T0200746

Statistical Development of Quality in Medicine

STATISTICS IN PRACTICE

Advisory Editor

Stephen Senn
University of Glasgow, UK

Founding Editor

Vic Barnett
Nottingham Trent University, UK

Statistics in Practice is an important international series of texts which provide detailed coverage of statistical concepts, methods and worked case studies in specific fields of investigation and study.

With sound motivation and many worked practical examples, the books show in down-to-earth terms how to select and use an appropriate range of statistical techniques in a particular practical field within each title's special topic area.

The books provide statistical support for professionals and research workers across a range of employment fields and research environments. Subject areas covered include medicine and pharmaceutics; industry, finance and commerce; public services; the earth and environmental sciences, and so on.

The books also provide support to students studying statistical courses applied to the above areas. The demand for graduates to be equipped for the work environment has led to such courses becoming increasingly prevalent at universities and colleges.

It is our aim to present judiciously chosen and well-written workbooks to meet everyday practical needs. Feedback of views from readers will be most valuable to monitor the success of this aim.

A complete list of titles in this series appears at the end of the volume.

Statistical Development of Quality in Medicine

Per Winkel
*Copenhagen Trial Unit, Centre for Clinical Intervention Research,
Rigshospitalet, Copenhagen University Hospital, Denmark*

Nien Fan Zhang
*US National Institute of Standards and Technology,
Gaithersburg, USA*

John Wiley & Sons, Ltd

Copyright © 2007   John Wiley & Sons Ltd, The Atrium, Southern Gate, Chichester,
West Sussex PO19 8SQ, England

Telephone (+44) 1243 779777

E-mail (for orders and customer service enquiries): cs-books@wiley.co.uk
Visit our Home Page on www.wileyeurope.com or www.wiley.com

All Rights Reserved. No part of this publication may be reproduced, stored in a retrieval system
or transmitted in any form or by any means, electronic, mechanical, photocopying, recording,
scanning or otherwise, except under the terms of the Copyright, Designs and Patents Act 1988
or under the terms of a licence issued by the Copyright Licensing Agency Ltd, 90 Tottenham
Court Road, London W1T 4LP, UK, without the permission in writing of the Publisher.
Requests to the Publisher should be addressed to the Permissions Department, John Wiley &
Sons Ltd, The Atrium, Southern Gate, Chichester, West Sussex PO19 8SQ, England, or emailed
to permreq@wiley.co.uk, or faxed to (+44) 1243 770620.

This publication is designed to provide accurate and authoritative information in regard to the
subject matter covered. It is sold on the understanding that the Publisher is not engaged in
rendering professional services. If professional advice or other expert assistance is required, the
services of a competent professional should be sought.

Other Wiley Editorial Offices

John Wiley & Sons Inc., 111 River Street, Hoboken, NJ 07030, USA

Jossey-Bass, 989 Market Street, San Francisco, CA 94103-1741, USA

Wiley-VCH Verlag GmbH, Boschstr. 12, D-69469 Weinheim, Germany

John Wiley & Sons Australia Ltd, 42 McDougall Street, Milton, Queensland 4064, Australia

John Wiley & Sons (Asia) Pte Ltd, 2 Clementi Loop #02-01, Jin Xing Distripark, Singapore
129809

John Wiley & Sons Canada Ltd, 6045 Freemont Blvd, Mississauga, ONT, L5R 4J3

Wiley also publishes its books in a variety of electronic formats. Some content that appears in
print may not be available in electronic books.

Anniversary Logo Design: Richard J. Pacifico

British Library Cataloguing in Publication Data

A catalogue record for this book is available from the British Library

ISBN- 13: 978-0-470-02777-6 (HB)

Typeset in 10.5/13 pt. Times by Thomson Digital
Printed and bound in Great Britain by TJ International, Padstow, Cornwall
This book is printed on acid-free paper responsibly manufactured from sustainable forestry
in which at least two trees are planted for each one used for paper production.

To my wife Hanne and my two sons Jon and Poul

PER WINKEL

To my wife Di Cheng Sun, our son Ning Zhang,
and our daughter Jing Yuan Zhang

NIEN FAN ZHANG

Contents

Preface

Our research collaboration started when Per Winkel was struggling with heavily autocorrelated laboratory quality control data. He contacted Nien Fan Zhang and asked for his help to solve the problems. The next time Per Winkel asked for Nien Fan Zhang's help was when planning to write an English textbook on statistical quality development in medicine. At that time Per Winkel had already written a Danish textbook on this topic [1]. Appendix A on basic statistics, and Chapters 1 and 2 on the theory of control charts and Shewhart charts have been translated from this book and subsequently reviewed and revised by Nien Fan Zhang to secure the statistical rigour. In addition to translating these chapters Per Winkel has added additional clinical examples to Chapters 1 and 2. But the English book needed to address the question on autocorrelated data and risk adjustment, which were only briefly mentioned in the Danish textbook. Since Nien Fan Zhang is doing active research within the areas of time-weighted control charts and control charts for autocorrelated data it was natural to ask Nien Fan Zhang to write the two Chapters, 3 Time-weighted control charts and 4 Control charts for autocorrelated data. In addition Nien Fan Zhang has written Appendix B, which contains a derivation of the control limits for $\overline{X}$ charts and S charts with unequal sample size, and Appendix C. Per Winkel has written the remaining chapters more directly related to clinical research, namely: the Introduction – on quality of health care in general, Chapter 1 Theory of statistical process control, Chapter 2 Shewhart control charts, Chapter 5 Tools of risk adjustment, Chapter 6 Risk-adjusted control charts, Chapter 7 Risk-adjusted comparison of healthcare providers, Chapter 8 Learning curves, and Chapter 9 Assessing the quality of clinical processes, as well as Appendix A. We have reviewed each other's chapters. During this process Nien Fan Zhang's main role, of course, has been to secure the statistical rigour and Per Winkel's to construct clinical examples when deemed necessary in order to ease understanding.

The purpose of this book is to present statistical techniques of major relevance for quality development in medicine. It is furnished with a collection of diverse examples of their application in clinical practice. The target group consists of people who are directly or indirectly involved in the quality assurance of clinical work, i.e., physicians, nurses, administrators, and students of topics related to medicine like epidemiology, bioengineering, etc. In terms of background statistical knowledge, the target group may be divided into three subgroups.

1. People with high school mathematics only.
2. People with basic statistical knowledge, e.g., acquired during post-graduate courses in applied statistics for nurses and physicians.
3. People with interest in quality assurance, epidemiology, etc. who are engaged in a more advanced statistical education.

The gap between group 1 and 2 may disappear because Appendix A, reviewing the basic statistical background of relevance for statistical process control (SPC), is included in the book. By studying the appendix, group 1 may reach the level of group 2. What is left then is to provide these two groups with:

a) The necessary understanding and command of basic statistical process control that enables them to identify practical quality assurance problems, which may be solved by using the SPC techniques, and subsequently to assess and apply relevant computer software to actually solve these problems.
b) Sufficient knowledge on the statistical techniques used in the scientific clinical literature on quality assurance. The target group then will be able to use clinical studies and critically assess the quality and limitation of the results.

For group 3, the book provide skills in using SPC in practice as well as an introduction to relevant statistical methods including diverse examples of their application within the field of clinical quality assurance. The book may then be used as an aid in conjunction with a more focused and advanced course in applied statistics, for instance in regression analysis and/or mixed model analysis.

It is always possible that errors may creep in while writing a book like this. Also we may have overlooked things that would have been relevant for inclusion. Therefore, we welcome any constructive criticism and suggestions for improvements of this book.

Acknowledgements

Our thanks are due to Christian Gluud who is the head of the Copenhagen Trial Unit, Centre for Clinical Intervention Research, Copenhagen University Hospital. His help during this work has been invaluable. From the start he has supported the project with great enthusiasm. He has reviewed all the chapters and his constructive criticism, overview of the clinical research literature, and suggestions for improvement of style, structure, and content have all been a tremendous help.

Our thanks are also due to Dimitrinka Nikolova for reviewing the style and language of the manuscript, to Styrbjørn Birch and Nader Salas for computer technical assistance as well other staff at the Copenhagen Trial Unit, Centre for Clinical Intervention Research, for providing friendly working conditions for Per Winkel.

Last but not least our thanks are due to Thomas Rump who allowed us to use the material from the Danish textbook [1].

REFERENCES

[1] Winkel P. Statistisk Kvalitetsudvikling i Klinik og Laboratorium. Ingeniørenlbøger, Ingeniøren A/S 2002.

Introduction – on Quality of Health Care in General

I.1 QUALITY OF HEALTH CARE

A concise, meaningful, and generally applicable definition of the quality of health care is difficult to give [1]. Donabedian [2] suggested that 'several formulations are both possible and legitimate, depending on where we are located in the system of care and on what the nature and extent of our responsibilities are'.

Healthcare professionals tend to define quality in terms of the care provided and received, and emphasise the technical quality and the interaction with the patient. The technical quality of care includes the appropriateness of the services provided and the skill with which appropriate care is performed. The quality of the interaction between physician and patient depends on the quality of their communication, the physician's ability to maintain the patient's trust, and treat the patient appropriately, i.e., showing concern, empathy, honesty, tact, and sensitivity [2]. There is a growing recognition that care must be responsive to the preferences and values of the consumers, in particular, individual patients. Therefore, the ability of the healthcare providers to meet the expectations of patients and other customers is an important quality parameter.

Another perspective is that of healthcare plans, organisations, and public agencies that purchase care for beneficiaries, e.g., a whole nation.

Statistical Development of Quality in Medicine   P. Winkel and N. F. Zhang
© 2007 John Wiley & Sons, Ltd

The emphasis here is on the enrolled population and attributes of care that reflect the functioning of the organisational systems, e.g., accessibility. The population-based perspective combined with the fact that resources are limited implies that the amount of care that some persons receive may be limited so that all members of the group receive the essential services.

A third perspective on quality is that of organised purchasers. Like the healthcare plans and public agencies they tend to be concerned with population-based measures of quality and organisational issues. Whether the interest of purchasers will conflict with the interests of patients is uncertain [1].

Three mechanisms have the potential to change the focus from the end-user of the healthcare system, namely the sick patient, to other issues and thus endanger the quality of care [3]:

1. If the risk of high, unanticipated costs for individual patients is not shared by a large organisation, but passed along to small groups of physicians or even individual physicians, the latter may find themselves in a situation where their financial interests and their loyalties to the patients are at conflict.
2. If the employers determine the details and limitations of the benefit package and their employees have no other choice, profit-maximisation may become an overriding issue.
3. If the focus shifts from the treatment of sick patients to the treatment of healthy individuals, the patient who needs the care may suffer. This may happen if the emphasis of a healthcare plan is on the health of the whole population of enrolees rather than the sick patients. For instance the availability of fitness programs may become a competition parameter.

I.2   MEASURES AND INDICATORS OF QUALITY OF HEALTH CARE

The quality of care can be evaluated on the basis of structure, process, and result. Structural data are the characteristics of physicians and hospitals. They could include a physician's specialty, the ownership of a hospital, availability of equipment, staffing levels, etc. Process data are the components of the encounter between a healthcare professional and a patient, for instance, the medication administered. A clinical process measure assesses performance based on adherence to established clinical standards. Throughput process measures are based on management data. They include such measures as waiting lists, ambulance response times, delays in emergency departments, etc. Result data include outcome data and costs incurred by producing a specified healthcare output. Outcome data refer to the patient's subsequent health status (e.g., improvement in mobility) and include observed outcomes, e.g., death, morbidity, and patient perceived outcomes such as satisfaction and quality of life.

To a large extent the clinical performance observed is a function of the clinical, organisational system in which individuals work rather than of a particular individual. Safety, patient satisfaction, surgical outcomes, infection rates, etc., are all linked to systems of information, architecture, scheduling, resource allocation, etc. Therefore, organisational quality measurement systems are more powerful in improving care than those that are individually focused. For instance, differences in structural factors (e.g., availability of equipment and staffing levels) are correlated with outcome [4]. Several institutional management processes have been found to be associated with improved outcomes in intensive care units [see 7].

It is important to make a distinction between a measure of quality and an indicator of quality. An example of a quality measure would be a clinical process measure based on agreed criteria supported by evidence or logic. For instance, avoiding delay in the use of antibiotics in pneumonia. A quality indicator would be, e.g., the death of a patient during a surgical procedure because the outcome is not only influenced by the quality of care but also by other factors, e.g., severity of disease, co-morbidity, the patient's socioeconomic status.

The focus of a quality measure or a quality indicator may be either on improving the quality of care or on aiding consumers in the selection of providers [5]. It is necessary not to confuse these two functions because they require very different formats.

I.3 THE FUNCTIONS OF QUALITY MEASURES AND INDICATORS

Any population evaluated, e.g., hospitals, healthcare groups, surgeons, will have a distribution of performance levels. The purpose of measuring this performance is to improve it. The goal may be accomplished in two ways that may or may not work in synergy: improvement through selection and improvement through changes in care [6].

I.3.1   Improvement through Selection

To improve the distribution of performance levels by selection the members of the population, i.e., the healthcare providers, must be made accountable. Therefore, the function of the quality measures and indicators in this case is to provide the users of healthcare providers with the information necessary to make an informed choice based on an assessment of the quality of the product they want to purchase. For a given user the quality indicator or measure must fulfil four criteria in order to be useful: (1) it must be relevant to the user's needs; for instance, a patient seeking the best preventive care may only be able to learn about mammography rates. (2) The ranking of the providers according to measurement value must correspond to a ranking according to the quality that the measurement portrays. (3) The measurement distribution must be current; for instance, surgical mortality figures that are five years old may very well be useless. (4) The data must be presented in a format that the user is able to understand.

I.3.1.1   Barriers to improvement through selection

There are several barriers to improvement through selection. The above requirements may not be fulfilled. The information available may not be relevant to the user, and the information may be difficult to understand. Furthermore, the users' belief that the quality may actually vary between healthcare providers may be weak; the performance benchmarks may be local, only reflecting the relative performance within a group of healthcare providers; and the consumer may not have the necessary background to comprehend the information. If the decision maker is not the primary user, the decision tends to be based on cost alone. For instance, managed-care plans involve an inherent conflict of interest. They pledge to take care of their enrolees, but their financial success depends on doing as little for them as possible [3].

Investments are required to improve report content and formatting and in particular to provide the users with the necessary skills and attitude to make informed decisions [6].

I.3.2   Improvement through Change

Improvement through selection does not require the participation of the healthcare providers. By contrast, improvement through change is only possible if they participate. In this context the quality measures and indicators are for internal use. But they may also in some cases provide useful information for the consumers. To be useful for the provider they should allow the latter to identify specific areas for improvement and to monitor the progress of quality improvement programs. This kind of data may or may not be suitable for public consumption as well. They are typically generated more often than data generated for consumption by entities external to the provider. They are usually more detailed and they may or may not contain information of relevance to the public. Data for accountability are usually summary statistics so far removed in time and so coarsely granulated that they contain little or no information useful for caregivers interested in improvement.

It is necessary that quality indicators can be used to identify specific areas that need improvement. Outcome measures like death rates or rates of morbidity lack this quality. For instance, variation in death rates depends on chance, which is quantifiable statistically, and it may depend on the quality of care. However, death rate is neither a sensitive nor a specific marker of quality of care with the possible exception of coronary artery bypass graft surgery [7]. The death rate namely depends on differences in the patient mixes in terms of severity of disease, co-morbidities, age, etc., and differences in definitions of the terms used to calculate the death rate as well as differences in the quality of the data. Case-mix differences may be adjusted for. But one never has any assurance that it works as intended [7, 8], and important risk factors may be unmeasured or unknown. Therefore, it is difficult to know what to do when outcome measures differ between healthcare institutions. Is it due to the use of different definitions, unsuccessful case-mix adjustment, structural factors such as differences in the ratio between physicians and patients, institutional management factors affecting clinical processes, clinical skill, or unknown clinical factors? Consequently, measurements of outcome data like death rates should only be made for research purposes or to detect extreme outliers [7]. By contrast, a strong case can be made in support of clinical process measures that are direct measures of performance based on adherence to established clinical standards [7, 9].

Several approaches to change are possible. Juran [10] has classified approaches to change into three categories: (1) methods that standardise and stabilise processes by making them well controlled (quality control), (2) changes that improve processes (reduce costs and/or increase performance) (quality improvement), and (3) design of totally new processes (quality design).

To improve performance the organisations and providers should have the ability to undertake systematic changes. This requires a reliable flow of useful information, education, and training in the techniques of process improvement; investment in time and change management to alter core work processes; alignment of organisational incentives with care improvement objectives; and leadership [6].

I.3.2.1 Barriers to improvement through change

A main barrier to improvement through change is a lack of organisational processes to support change [6]. Contradictory incentives and failed integration is stalling progress. Most healthcare systems comprise a loose confederation of institutions that barely communicate. This type of organisation motivates each unit within the confederation to maximise its own return and often to work at cross-purposes with other entities.

Another main barrier is lack of investment in information systems that will collect data across settings, support efforts to understand patterns of care, and improve them and contribute to externally-required reporting [6]. The investment required may well be beyond the capacity of many small and midsized health systems. Furthermore, the absence of industry-wide standards is an important discouraging factor.

REFERENCES

[1] Blumenthal D. Quality of care – what is it? (Part one of six). N Eng J Med 1996; 335:891–4.

[2] Donabedian A. The quality of care: how can it be assessed? JAMA 1988; 260: 1743–8.

[3] Angell M, Kassirer JP. Quality and the medical marketplace – following elephants. N Engl J Med 1996; 335:883–5.

[4] Aiken LH, Clarke SP, Sloane DM, Sochalski J, Silber JH. Hospital nurse staffing and patient mortality, nurse burnout, and job dissatisfaction. JAMA 2002; 288:1984–8.

[5] Press I. The measure of quality. Q Manage Health Care 2004; 13:202–9.

[6] Berwick DM, James B, Coye MJ. Connections between quality measurement and improvement. Med Care 2003; 41(1 suppl):I30–8.

[7] Lilford R, Mohammed MA, Spiegelhalter D, Thomsom R. Use and misuse of process and outcome data in managing performance of acute medical care: avoiding institutional stigma. Lancet 2004; 363:1147–54.

[8] Deeks JJ, Dinnes J, D'Amico R, Sowden AJ, Sakarovitch C, Song F, Petticrew M, Altman DG. Evaluating non-randomized intervention studies. Health Technol Assess 2003; 7:1–186.

[9] Kurstein P, Gluud LL, Willemann M, Olsen KR, Kjellberg J, Sogaard J, Gluud C. Agreement between reported use of interventions for liver diseases and research evidence in Cochrane systematic reviews. J Hepatol 2005; 43:984–9.
[10] Juran JM, ed. Juran's Quality Control Handbook, 4th Edition. McGraw-Hill, New York, 1988.

Part I

Control Charts

1

Theory of Statistical Process Control

The most important tool in statistical process control is the control chart. Shewhart developed the first type of chart during the 1920s [1]. One of the most commonly used Shewhart charts is the $\overline{X}$ chart. In the following for illustration, we will use this chart. However, the principles reviewed may be broadened without much effort to include control charts in general.

Originally control charts were developed in order to solve industrial problems. We will start with pharmaceutical examples followed by applications within the health care sector. The analogies and differences between industrial and healthcare problems are also discussed.

1.1 STATISTICAL FOUNDATION OF CONTROL CHARTS

To characterise a process, products produced by the process may be sampled. A process variable is a random variable which value is obtained by observing or measuring a specified property of each product, produced by the process and reflecting its quality. A sample variable is also a random variable. However, its value is calculated as a function of the process variable values, measured in the sample.

Statistical Development of Quality in Medicine   P. Winkel and N. F. Zhang
© 2007 John Wiley & Sons, Ltd

Sample values are used to construct a control chart. They are subsequently plotted on the chart to monitor the process.

1.1.1 Statistical Control

Statistical control is a concept fundamental to the theory of control charts. It is based on a distinction between two types of variation: one resulting from unavoidable causes, which one cannot identify (random variation), and one resulting from causes, which may be identified (assignable causes of variation). A process which sample values vary due to random causes alone is said to be in a state of statistical control. Additional variation caused by assignable causes may occur. If this is the case, the process is said to be out of statistical control. Since these causes may be identified, it is often possible to regulate and control them so that the process may be brought back into a state of statistical control.

Although the causes of variation of sample values from a process in statistical control cannot be identified, the type and extent of the variation may be described using large volumes of data. In other words, the values may be described approximately by a probability distribution. The parameters of this distribution characterise the state of the process. Information about this probability distribution may be obtained from random samples selected from the process while it is in statistical control.

1.1.2 Samples and Control Charts

Assume we are examining the production process for a pharmaceutical product (e.g., tablets) that is in statistical control. The machine producing the tablets has been adjusted to produce tablets with a weight that follows a Gaussian distribution with a mean of 63.000 mg and a standard deviation of 0.010 mg. Samples, each comprising one tablet, are selected from the production batch and their weights measured. We assume the error of measurement is negligible and that the machine is functioning as anticipated. Therefore, the results of the measurements follow a Gaussian distribution with mean 63.000 mg and standard deviation 0.010 mg. In the long run, we expect 99.73 % of the results to fall within an interval with its upper limit equal to the mean plus three standard deviations and the lower one equal to the mean minus three standard deviations, i.e., an interval between 62.970 mg and 63.030 mg (see Appendix A, Example A.11). The distribution with these limits entered is depicted in Figure 1.1 a.

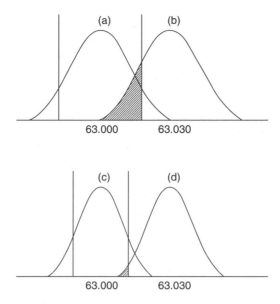

Figure 1.1 The distribution of the sample mean of the weight of tablets before ((a) and (c)) and after ((b) and (d)) the adjustment of a tablet-producing machine has been changed by 0.030 mg. Figures (a) and (b) show the distributions for sample size − 1 and figures (c) and (d) the distributions when the sample size = 2.

Had we selected samples comprising not one, but n $(n > 1)$ tablets, it would have been natural to calculate the mean of the n measurement results if we wanted to follow the mean value of the process. The distribution of the weight is Gaussian. The mean of the results of n measurements generated by this distribution also follows a Gaussian distribution with the same mean, but with a standard deviation of $\frac{\sigma}{\sqrt{n}}$ (see Appendix A, Equation (A.23)). We may, therefore, calculate an interval within which 99.73 % of the sample means will fall in the long run. The lower limit of this interval is $\mu - \frac{3\sigma}{\sqrt{n}}$, and its upper limit is $\mu + \frac{3\sigma}{\sqrt{n}}$, i.e., $63.000 - \frac{3 \cdot 0.010}{\sqrt{n}}$ mg and $63.000 + \frac{3 \cdot 0.010}{\sqrt{n}}$ mg, respectively.

Figure 1.1 (a) depicts the distribution with these limits calculated for $n = 1$, and Figure 1.1 (c) depicts the distribution with the limits calculated for $n = 2$. Both of the intervals include 99.73 % of all values. However, the interval for the mean values ($n = 2$) is slimmer than that for the single values ($n = 1$) because it has a smaller standard deviation.

Now, assume that the machine is adjusted so that the mean value of the weight of tablets is increased by 0.030 mg. It will continue to produce tablets, the weights of which follow a Gaussian distribution with standard deviation 0.010 mg. However, the mean has increased to 63.030 mg. The distribution of single values (see Figure 1.1 (b)) as well as the distribution of sample means (see Figure 1.1 (d)) will change. In both cases the distribution will be horizontally shifted towards the right so that the mean value now will be 63.030 mg instead of 63.000 mg. After the mean value of the process has changed, a large proportion of the sample values (single values for $n = 1$ and mean values for $n = 2$) will fall outside the upper limit in both cases. However, some of them will still fall within the two limits (the control limits). The proportion falling within the control limits will be larger when the sample size is 1 than when it is 2. This is so because the two distributions before and after the shift of the mean value of the process are slimmer and therefore better separated when the sample size is 2 than when it is 1.

We will now construct a control chart. To do so we rotate Figure 1.1 (c) 90° counter clockwise and draw four horizontal lines passing through zero, the lower control limit, the process mean, and the upper control limit, respectively. The line passing through zero is used to indicate the time or the order of the samples. The result is depicted in Figure 1.2.

The fraction of a Gaussian distribution, with mean μ and standard deviation σ, that is delimited by the values $\mu \pm 3\sigma$, is 99.73 % and the remaining fraction located outside the interval is 100 % − 99.73 % = 0.27 %. Therefore, the probability that a sample mean falls outside the $(\mu \pm \frac{3\sigma}{\sqrt{n}})$ limits of a control chart is 0.27 %, as long as the process remains in statistical control. Each time we select a sample, we test the null hypothesis that the mean value of the process has not changed by checking if the sample mean falls within or outside the control limits given above. The level of significance of this test is 100 % − 99.73 % = 0.27 %. It follows that the control chart may be used repeatedly to test the hypothesis that the process is in statistical control. It is implicitly assumed that the value of σ never changes.

Example 1.1

A sample comprising five tablets is selected each day from a process producing tablets, and the weight of each tablet is measured. The mean value of the results of the measurements is calculated. The mean value and standard deviation of the process are known to be 63.000 mg and 0.010 mg, respectively. We want to construct a control chart with control limits equal to the mean ±3 standard deviations of the sample mean. Because the

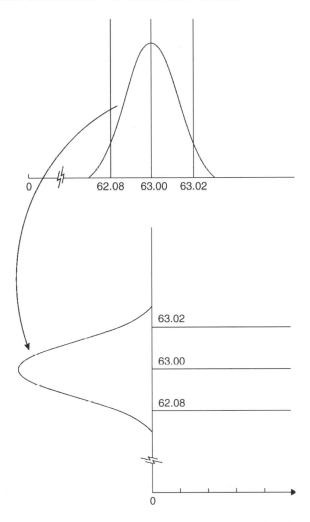

Figure 1.2 The construction of a control chart based on the distribution shown in Figure 1.1 (c). The distribution has been rotated 90 degrees counter clockwise. The line corresponding to the mean value is the centreline, and the lines corresponding to the limits of the 99.73 % confidence interval are the control limits of the chart.

sample size, n, is 5, the standard deviation of $\bar{x}$ (the sample mean) is: $\frac{0.010}{\sqrt{5}} = 0.0045$ mg (see Appendix A, Equation (A.23)). The mean of the distribution of sample means is the same as that of the process, i.e., 63.000 mg. The centreline of the chart, therefore, is at 63.000 mg. The upper and lower control limits are $63.000 + 3 \cdot 0.0045 = 63.035$ mg and $63.000 - 3 \cdot 0.0045 = 62.986$ mg, respectively.

In the above it has been assumed that the process has been so well described that its parameters may be considered known. As a rule this is not so, and we have to use estimates of the parameters when constructing a control chart.

1.2 USE OF CONTROL CHARTS

Initially, when one constructs a control chart, it is usually not known if the process is in statistical control. In the initial phase the goal is to reduce the variation of the process until it reaches a state of statistical control that is acceptable. To assess if a process is in statistical control, one often uses 20 to 25 samples, each comprising 4 to 5 observations. When the samples are collected, one should record those conditions that might possibly create variation in addition to the random variation. This could be, e.g., the temperature, the raw materials used, the identity of operators, etc. The average of the individual sample means ($\hat{\mu}$) is used as an estimate of the mean of the process variable. It defines the location of the centreline. An unbiased estimate of the process standard deviation ($\hat{\sigma}$) is calculated from the average of the standard deviations (s_i) of the individual samples ($\bar{s}$) divided by a factor (c_4), which depends of the sample size and is found using Table 1.1.

We have

$$\hat{\mu} = \frac{\sum_{i=1}^{k} \bar{x}_i}{k} \tag{1.1}$$

where k is the number of samples and

$$\hat{\sigma} = \frac{\bar{s}}{c_4} = \frac{\sum_{i=1}^{k} s_i}{k \cdot c_4} \tag{1.2}$$

The upper control limit (UCL) is calculated as

$$\text{UCL} = \hat{\mu} + 3 \frac{\hat{\sigma}}{\sqrt{n}} \tag{1.3}$$

and the lower control limit (LCL) as

$$\text{LCL} = \hat{\mu} - 3 \frac{\hat{\sigma}}{\sqrt{n}} \tag{1.4}$$

Table 1.1 Factors used for $\overline{X}$ charts and/or S charts.

Sample size	Factors				
n	c_4	B_3	B_4	B_5	B_6
2	0.7979	0.000	3.267	0.000	2.606
3	0.8862	0.000	2.568	0.000	2.276
4	0.9213	0.000	2.266	0.000	2.088
5	0.9400	0.000	2.089	0.000	1.964
6	0.9515	0.030	1.970	0.029	1.874
7	0.9594	0.118	1.882	0.113	1.806
8	0.9650	0.185	1.815	0.179	1.751
9	0.9693	0.239	1.761	0.232	1.707
10	0.9727	0.284	1.716	0.276	1.669
11	0.9754	0.321	1.679	0.313	1.637
12	0.9776	0.354	1.646	0.346	1.610
13	0.9794	0.382	1.618	0.374	1.585
14	0.9810	0.406	1.594	0.399	1.563
15	0.9823	0.428	1.572	0.421	1.544
16	0.9835	0.448	1.552	0.440	1.526
17	0.9845	0.466	1.534	0.458	1.511
18	0.9854	0.482	1.518	0.475	1.496
19	0.9862	0.497	1.503	0.490	1.483
20	0.9869	0.510	1.490	0.504	1.470
21	0.9876	0.523	1.477	0.516	1.459
22	0.9882	0.534	1.466	0.528	1.448
23	0.9887	0.545	1.455	0.539	1.438
24	0.9892	0.555	1.445	0.549	1.429
25	0.9896	0.565	1.435	0.559	1.420

For $n > 25$, $c_4 \approx \dfrac{4(n-1)}{4n-3}$

where n is the sample size. Finally, the individual sample mean values are depicted on the chart. In the case where all points lie within the control limits, the data are consistent with the hypothesis that the process is in statistical control. If one or more points are located outside the limits, it is an indication that the process is not in statistical control, and the causes must be traced. In the cases where these causes are identified, the corresponding values are eliminated from the calculations, and a revised control chart is computed. It is now controlled if all of the remaining points fall within the revised control limits. Since the revised control limits are narrower than the original ones, data points that previously fell within the original limits may now fall outside the revised limits. The cause, why a point fell outside the limits, may not necessarily be found. If this is the case for only one or few points, one may choose not to remove the values immediately, but wait and see how the control chart functions and eventually remove them later on. If a large number of points are falling outside the limits for unknown reasons, the pattern formed by the points should be inspected. By doing so, one may often be able to identify a cause common to all points. After a while, hopefully, the chart indicates that a state consistent with the hypothesis of statistical control has been reached. If the level of the process and the variation relative to this level are both acceptable, the chart specifies the objective of the process.

At this stage, it is vitally important that a protocol is written specifying how one should go about looking for special causes if a value falls outside the control limits, and how the report resulting from such a search should be made. The specifics of the protocol depend on the process. For a good clinical example see [2]. The chart may, then, be used to monitor regularly selected samples, the mean values of which are depicted on the chart. As long as these values are located within the control limits, one may assume that the process is in statistical control. The data cumulated in this way may be used to calculate relatively precise estimates of the parameters of the process. When reliable estimates are available, one may determine if the process actually meets the quality requirements. If this is not the case, it is advisable to revise the process, i.e., to improve it, until it meets the demands. In this phase statistical design of exploratory experiments is an important tool. A review of these techniques, however, is outside the scope of this book. The interested reader is referred to [3].

Example 1.2

At an outpatient clinic the management decided to take random samples comprising 30 ambulatory patients on each weekday for four weeks to study the patient waiting times and assess if the quality requirement for patient waiting times was met. The employees at the clinic were not aware of this investigation. The waiting time of each patient was recorded. A patient's waiting time is the period starting when the patient arrives at the clinic and ending when a technologist sees the patient. Thus, 20 samples each comprising 30 randomly selected waiting times were recorded.

Table 1.2 The mean and standard deviation of waiting times (minutes from patient's arrival at outpatient clinic until seen by a technologist) recorded on each of 20 weekdays.

Sample #	n	$\bar{x}$	$\bar{s}$
1	30	16.75	5.509
2	30	15.60	4.558
3	30	16.14	5.465
4	30	15.96	4.582
5	30	18.86	4.594
6	30	14.33	4.920
7	30	15.44	6.357
8	30	14.67	3.791
9	30	16.53	6.885
10	30	19.89	5.583
11	30	14.37	3.714
12	30	14.13	3.477
13	30	14.99	4.627
14	30	13.33	3.922
15	30	19.96	4.717
16	30	15.87	5.481
17	30	14.41	5.877
18	30	15.16	4.901
19	30	13.82	5.434
20	30	18.46	3.716
		$\hat{\mu} = 15.93$	$s = 4.905$
			$\hat{\sigma} = 4.95$

Table 1.2 shows the 20 sample mean values and standard deviations. The mean of the mean values ($\hat{\mu} = 15.93$ minute) estimating the process mean and the average of the standard deviations ($\bar{s} = 4.905$ minute) are also shown. An unbiased estimate of the process standard deviation ($\hat{\sigma}$) is calculated by dividing $\bar{s}$ by c_4. The latter quantity is calculated as $\frac{4(30-1)}{120-3} = 0.9915$ (see Table 1.1). Therefore, $\hat{\sigma}$ is $\frac{4.905}{0.9915} = 4.95$ minute. Using these data an $\overline{X}$ control chart may be constructed. The estimate of the standard deviation of the sample mean values is $\frac{4.95}{\sqrt{30}} = 0.90$ minute since the sample size is 30. The centreline of the $\overline{X}$ chart is at 15.9 minute ($\hat{\mu}$), the UCL is $15.9 + 3 \cdot 0.90 = 18.6$ minute, and the LCL is $15.9 - 3 \cdot 0.90 = 13.2$ minute.

Figure 1.3 (a) shows the $\overline{X}$ chart. The sample means are depicted on the chart. Since three of the values (samples # 5, # 10, and # 15) are located above the UCL, the process is not in statistical control.

Figure 1.3 (b) shows a revised control chart after these three values have been eliminated from the calculations. Now the last value is outside the UCL. Figure 1.3 (c) shows the control chart calculated without using

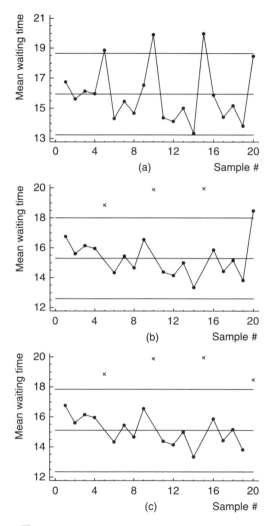

Figure 1.3   (a) An $\overline{X}$ chart showing the mean waiting times (minute) on weekdays. (b) The control chart shown in (a) after the results of samples # 5, # 10, and # 15 have been removed and the chart calculated without using these values. The latter values are depicted as crosses. (c) The control chart shown in (a), after the results of samples # 5, # 10, # 15, and # 20 have been removed and the chart calculated without using these values. The latter values are depicted as crosses.

this value. The chart is consistent with a process in statistical control. The management now had two jobs. First the special cause of the excess variation had to be found and removed and the process brought into a state of statistical control. Then the estimated process parameters had to be compared with the quality requirements for waiting times to assess the quality of the process.

Inspecting the pattern of values (# 5, # 10, # 15, and # 20) outside the UCL, one notes that all values were collected on a Friday. It turned out that on Fridays the patient mix differed from that of the other weekdays in that an unusually large number of patients from the cardiology department were scheduled for ECG recordings in addition to blood specimen collection. These patients required more time than those not scheduled for ECG recordings. A retrospective analysis revealed that overtime was much more common on Fridays than on any other weekday. To prepare the organisation for quality assessment and control on a routine basis, the management purchased a system for automatic recording of waiting times. The IDs of technologists doing venipunctures and recording ECGs were already automatically captured by the current clinical data processing system. We will return to this example in Chapter 9.

Table 1.3 shows the protocol they designed for the search for special causes to be used when the process was brought into a state of statistical control of a sufficiently high quality.

Table 1.3 Procedure for tracking special cause variation. Start at step 0 and proceed to the right.

Step	Actions	Questions and routing in table	
0	Control data and data processing.	Can error in data explain variation?	If yes, go to step 4. If no, go to step 1.
1	Compute ECG in number of venipuncture equivalents. Express production in number of venipunctures. Control staffing of ambulatory.	Can increased production or decreased staffing explain variation?	If no go to step 2. If yes, go to step 4.
2	Define productivity as venipuncture/technologist hour. Compute 1) average productivity, 2) average productivity per 30 minute period, 3) average productivity per technologist, and 4) average productivity per technologist per 30 minute period. Identify significantly outlying values.		Go to step 3.
3	Interview manager of ambulatory and technologists.		Go to step 4.
4	Write report and stop.		

1.3 DESIGN OF CONTROL CHARTS

When one constructs a control chart, it is necessary to decide which control limits, sample size, and sampling frequency one wants to use.

1.3.1 Control Limits

Clearly, the position of the control limits has a bearing on the function of a control chart. The further away from the centreline the limits are located, the fewer sample means will fall outside the limits. This implies that the probability that a type-1 error will be committed declines. A type-1 error is committed when a sample mean value falls outside the control limits even though the process is in statistical control. It is then assumed that the process is out of statistical control, and a search for the cause is initiated. The price of decreasing the expected number of type-1 errors, by widening the limits, is an increase in the expected number of type-2 errors. A type-2 error is committed if a sample mean value falls within the control limits and thereby prevents one from acknowledging that the process is no longer in statistical control. If one narrows the limits, the probability of committing a type-2 error declines, but at the same time that of committing a type-1 error increases.

The choice of control limits depends on a weighing of the pros and cons of the two types of errors. One approach is to decide initially how large a fraction (α) of the sample means one is willing to let fall outside the limits, while the process is in statistical control. The position of the control limits is then calculated so that this condition is fulfilled. If the fraction of values falling outside the limits is α, the fraction of values falling within the limits must be $(1 - \alpha)$. In the case of the $\overline{X}$ chart, the problem may be stated as follows: We need to find a number, k, so that the probability that a sample mean will fall inside the control limits is

$$P\left(\mu - \frac{k\sigma}{\sqrt{n}} \leq \overline{X} \leq \mu + \frac{k\sigma}{\sqrt{n}}\right) = 1 - \alpha \qquad (1.5)$$

where μ is the mean of the process, σ its standard deviation, $\overline{X}$ the sample mean, and n the sample size. It is not particularly difficult to find k in Equation (1.5) when the distribution of $\overline{X}$ is Gaussian and μ and σ are both known. When the value of k has been determined in this way, the UCL is set equal to $\mu + \frac{k\sigma}{\sqrt{n}}$, and the LCL is set equal to $\mu - \frac{k\sigma}{\sqrt{n}}$. Usually $k = 3$ is used. Inserting this value in Equation (1.5) the corresponding value of α may be calculated. One finds that $\alpha = 0.0027$. Therefore, in the long run, $(1 - 0.0027)100\,\% = 99.73\,\%$ of the sample mean values will fall within the limits, as long as the process remains in statistical control. In the following we will use the factor 3, when calculating control limits. It is assumed that the sample mean follows a Gaussian distribution and the parameters are known. Due to the central limit theorem (see Appendix A, Section A.3.4.1), the assumption of a Gaussian distribution is not necessary when the sample size is large enough.

In addition to the control limits, two warning limits are sometimes used, one on each side of the centreline usually at a distance of two standard deviations from it. If a sample value falls between a warning limit and the corresponding control limit, then it is a warning that the process may be out of statistical control.

It is not always safe to assume that a sample variable follows a Gaussian distribution, as we have done previously. However, the consequences of erroneously making this assumption are limited. This appears from an improvement on Tchebichev's inequality [4], which may be phrased as follows: If the statistical variable X follows a unimodal distribution whose mode is equal to the mean, the probability that its value deviates from the distribution's mean value by more than k times its standard deviation is equal to or less than $\frac{1}{2.25k^2}$. A unimodal distribution is defined as a probability distribution which density function decreases monotonously to the left, as well as the right of its mode (see Appendix A, Section A.2.3). Based on the inequality above, for $k = 3$ the probability that a sample mean falls outside the control limits is $\frac{1}{2.25 \cdot 3^2} = 0.049$, or less, as long as the distribution of the sample mean is unimodal, and its mode and mean coincide.

1.3.2   Sample Size

If a process gets out of statistical control because its level is changing, the probability that a sample mean assumes a value outside the limits whereby the change will be acknowledged increases. The increase in probability depends on the sample size, as illustrated in Figure 1.1 in Section 1.1.2. The figure shows the distribution of the sample value before and after the mean has changed for sample size equal to 1 (upper frame) and for sample size equal to 2 (lower frame). When the sample size is 1, a much smaller fraction of the horizontally shifted distribution falls outside the control limits of the original distribution than in the case when the sample size is 2. Therefore, the probability (the area outside the control limits) that a specified change in the mean is acknowledged is smaller with sample size of 1 than with 2.

1.3.3 Sampling Frequency

The more frequently samples are selected, the sooner a change of the level of the process will be acknowledged; but also, the more frequently a sample mean value will fall outside the control limits while the process is in statistical control.

1.4 RATIONAL SAMPLES

A key issue to the construction of control charts is the formation of rational samples. Rational samples are composed so that assignable causes of variation may influence the variation between samples, but not the variation within samples. For instance, it will be inexpedient to mix the blood smears from two different technologists in the same sample because variation caused by differences between the two technologists will then not be acknowledged. The formation of rational samples is crucial and often requires considerable knowledge about the process in question.

If a process is in statistical control, all of the variation between the sample mean values can be explained by the variation within the samples because the process mean does not change. Therefore, the samples may be pooled and all be used to calculate a single estimate of the standard deviation. However, if the process is not in statistical control, the process mean may change between samples. In this case the standard deviation obtained by pooling the values will be larger than the standard deviation that one would obtain by calculating the average of the within-samples standard deviations. Since it is not known in advance whether a process is in statistical control, the average of the sample standard deviations should always be used. Otherwise the risk is that a lack of statistical control may be masked.

1.5 ANALYSING THE PROPERTIES OF A CONTROL CHART

Once a process is brought into a state of statistical control, a control chart may be used to monitor it. The purpose is to recognise quickly and in an objective way if the process gets out of statistical control. If a sample value falls outside the control limits, it is a very strong indication that this has happened. However, the values may remain within the control limits, while the process is out of control. A state of statistical control is characterised by control values scattering at random around the centreline. Therefore, if systematic sequences of values begin to appear, it may be an indication that the process is out of control, even though all values stay within the limits. A sequence of values that all share the same quality is referred to as a run. Eight consecutive sample mean values, each being larger than its predecessor, or eight values all located on the same side of the centreline are examples of runs.

To better characterise the values entered on the chart, it is customary to enter two warning limits; a lower one and an upper one. As mentioned previously, each of them is located at a distance of two standard deviations from the centreline. The probability that a sample mean value falls outside the warning limits is approximately 0.05 if the process is in control. However, the probability that two mean values in a row fall outside the upper warning limit is quite low. Therefore, this indicates strongly that the mean value of the process has increased. The two warning limits may be supplemented by an additional pair of warning limits located on each side of the centreline, each at a distance of one standard deviation from the line. In this way, the region defined by the two control limits is divided into 6 zones. This makes it easier to recognise interesting runs, e.g., a run characterised by values located above the same inner warning limit.

1.5.1 Systematic Data Patterns

We may test statistically if it is improbable that a run is just a random phenomenon. Then, it may be concluded that the process is out of statistical control. However, if one applies several tests simultaneously, i.e., pays attention to many different types of runs, the combined probability of committing a type-1 error may be quite high. Therefore, it is not recommendable routinely to include tests based on various types of runs when assessing whether a process is in statistical control or not. Small changes of the mean level may certainly cause various types of runs to appear while all data points are still falling within the control limits. However, to identify small changes in the level, it is recommended instead to apply a time-weighted control chart. These control charts are reviewed in Chapter 3. This is not to say that one should not pay attention to extreme patterns and utilise the information thus gained. When a value falls outside the control limits, statistically significant patterns of runs may be valuable clues in the search for the cause of the loss of control.

1.5.2　In-Control Average Run Length (ARL) and Out-of-Control ARL

In the following a process is considered to be in statistical control as long as the sample mean value stays within the control limits and out of control if a value falls outside the control limits. This usage of the chart implies that one is currently testing the hypothesis that the process is in control. Since the conclusions drawn on the basis of a statistical test result are inherently uncertain, one will occasionally commit an error. It is of practical interest to know how often one should expect a false alarm and thereby be led to commit a type-1 error. It is furthermore of interest to know the length of the period, from a loss of statistical control until the loss is acknowledged. The last question cannot be answered unequivocally unless it is specified how much out of control the process is in terms of the magnitude of the change of its parameter values.

The probability distribution of the sample means after the mean value of the process has changed is Gaussian with a mean equal to the new process mean value and a standard deviation equal to that characterising the distribution prior to the change. Using this information, one may calculate the fraction of the distribution delimited by the control limits (see Figure 1.1). This fraction is equal to the probability (β) that a sample mean will fall within the control limits and thereby prevent the change from being acknowledged. The probability that the mean value of the first sample selected – subsequent to a specified change of the process mean – falls outside the control limits is $1 - \beta$. This follows because β is the probability that it falls within the limits. The probability that the change will be acknowledged when the second sample is selected, is the probability (β) that it will not be acknowledged when the first sample is selected multiplied by the probability $(1 - \beta)$ that it will be when the second sample is selected, i.e., $\beta(1 - \beta)$. It is assumed that the sample values are statistically independent. The probability that the change will be acknowledged when the fifth sample is selected is $\beta^4(1 - \beta)$, etc. In general we have, that the probability that the change will be acknowledged at the kth trial is $\beta^{k-1}(1 - \beta)$. In the first example, it was necessary to obtain 2 samples before the change was acknowledged, and in the second example it was necessary to obtain 5 samples. To calculate the average number of samples necessary to select before a specified change is acknowledged, each possible outcome should be weighted by its probability of taking place and the resulting products added. In principle, there are an infinite number of possible outcomes, and the sum, therefore, includes an infinite number of terms. It may be shown that the sum is $\frac{1}{1-\beta}$. We have

$$\sum_{k=1}^{\infty} k\beta^{k-1}(1-\beta) = \frac{1}{1-\beta} \tag{1.6}$$

In the special case when the process mean has not changed, $(1-\beta)$, the probability that a value falls outside the control limits is equal to α, the risk of committing a type-1 error. The average number of samples collected (ARL, the average run length) between type-1 errors is called the in-control ARL. According to Equation (1.6) it is calculated as

$$\text{ARL}_\alpha = \frac{1}{\alpha} \tag{1.7}$$

Example 1.3

Using the conventional control limits equal to the process mean ± 3 standard deviations implies that $\alpha = 0.0027$. Therefore, the $\text{ARL}_{0.0027}$ between type-1 errors is $\frac{1}{0.0027} = 370.37$, according to Equation (1.7).

When β is known, Equation (1.6) may be used to calculate the average number of samples selected subsequent to a specified change of the process mean and before the first value falls outside the limits and the change thereby is acknowledged. We have

$$\text{ARL}_\beta = \frac{1}{1-\beta} \tag{1.8}$$

1.6 CHECKLISTS AND PARETO CHARTS

Two helpful instruments may supplement a control chart: a checklist and a Pareto chart. A checklist is used to list in a chronological order the problems that one has come across so far while monitoring the process. It should include information about how often the various flaws and defects have been observed and who took care of them. A Pareto chart

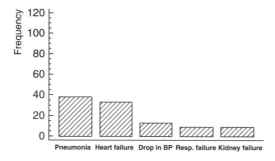

Figure 1.4 A Pareto chart showing the occurrence of postoperative medical complications in 102 surgical patients. BP stands for blood pressure, and Resp. stands for respiratory.

is in many ways similar to a histogram. The ordinate of a Pareto chart is the same, i.e., frequency. The abscissa, however, is qualitative instead of quantitative. It shows the type of problems one has come across. The chart gives a graphical representation of qualitative data, with the frequencies sorted according to size. The checklist may be used as input for the Pareto chart. The chart may be used to identify frequently occurring problems. However, it does not acknowledge the seriousness of the various problems. If some problems are serious and other problems are trivial ones, one might weigh the frequencies of the various problems according to their seriousness before drawing the Pareto chart.

Example 1.4

In each of 102 surgical patients the complications arising during the operation were noted. Figure 1.4 shows a Pareto chart of the frequencies of the various types of medical complications. It appears that heart failure and infection of the lungs are the predominant medical complications.

1.7   CLINICAL APPLICATIONS OF CONTROL CHARTS

The clinical applications of control charts are often less straightforward than the industrial ones. We will discuss the problems arising. Some of the issues will be further elaborated in Chapter 6.

1.7.1 Input/Output of Clinical Processes

In principle control charts may be used in clinical work in the same way as they are used in industrial work. The values of quality measures or quality indicators are measured as mentioned in the introduction and used to construct control charts. The quality may then be assessed and monitored using the charts.

The input to industrial processes may be controlled. However, this is not always the case for medical processes. In clinical medicine the patients vary considerably. Some patients may be so sick that they will not survive even if the clinical process, i.e., treatment and care, is optimal, while other patients whose diseases are less severe may survive even though the treatment and care they receive is of a poor quality. An industrial concern is able to standardise the input to its various processes. Therefore, one may safely assume that variation of the output (the products) mirrors the quality of the processes. By contrast, a hospital department or a practice cannot control the input (the number and types of patients received). Therefore, in this case, it is necessary to separate the variation of the output into two components: one that is caused by variation of the input (variation of severity of the patients' diseases, their co-morbidities, etc.) and one that is caused by the process (treatment and care). The problem may be dealt with in various ways as will be explained in Chapters 5, 6, and 7.

1.7.2 Samples

If possible, the samples formed should be rational. Therefore, assignable causes of variation should not be allowed to influence the within sample variation, and the selection of samples should be organised so that rational hypotheses of interest may be tested. Assume, e.g., that there are reasons to believe that the waiting-time between the arrival of a test request to a laboratory and the reporting of the corresponding result is not the same during working hours, as it is outside working hours. To assess this hypothesis, it is necessary to select 'waiting-time samples' so that a sample is either selected during working hours or outside working hours and not just at random times round the clock.

Two principles may be applied to form rational samples. According to one principle a sample should only include products that are produced at the same time (or as close together in time as possible). This principle is applied when the primary purpose is to be able to acknowledge a change in the process mean since the likelihood that such a change will affect the within-sample variation is very small. According to the other principle, the sampling period is extended. At the end of one sampling period, the next one is initiated, etc. Each sample consists of products representative of those produced since the last sample was selected. This principle is usually applied when a decision has to be made as to whether or not the products produced during the sampling period should be accepted. Supporters of the last principle often emphasise that a shift in the level, away from the control level and back again, in between sampling will not be acknowledged if the first principle is applied. However, if the process mean value fluctuates among different levels during the sampling period, the variation within the sample might be quite large. Therefore, it is possible to make any process look as if it were in control simply by lengthening the sampling period. In medicine all information about each patient is kept. Therefore, it makes sense to inspect all of the production. This implies that the second principle should be applied. Consequently, the samples should be as small as possible so that the conditions during the sampling are reasonably uniform. This also allows the search for the reason why a process is out of control to be conducted, while the trail is 'still hot'. Furthermore, actions necessary to remove the cause of a lack of statistical control will not be unduly delayed. For example we would want to detect an increase in the occurrence of Methicillin resistant *Staphylococcus aureus* infections as soon as possible to take the necessary precautions. On the other hand, the event one monitors (e.g., that a patient dies) may be a rare one. This requires the sample of patients to be made sufficiently large so that at least a few dead patients are included in each patient group. There are several considerations that one has to balance relative to each other before the sample size is decided.

Instead of using equally sized samples, it may be more practical to use equally sized sampling periods, e.g., a week, a month, or a quarter of a year. This implies that the sample size will vary. The above considerations then have to be balanced when the length of the sampling period is decided.

1.8 INAPPROPRIATE CHANGES OF A PROCESS

If the quality of a clinical process is not good enough for its purpose it has to be improved. To improve the quality of a process one has to change it. However, it is important to know when it is appropriate to change a process and when it is not. A process in statistical control may be changed if its quality is deemed insufficient for its purpose on the basis of an assessment of its parameter values. However, it should not be changed on the basis of an assessment of a sample obtained from it. If the system is not in statistical control it should not be changed. The reason is that the results of a change cannot usually be interpreted. Instead, the process should be brought into a state of statistical control and then changed if deemed necessary.

We will present an example illustrating the effect of using sample values as a basis for changing a system that is in statistical control and examples showing the effect of changing a system that is not in statistical control.

1.8.1 Changing a Process in Statistical Control Guided by Samples

Example 1.5

Table 1.4 (column 2) shows a series of 15 numbers drawn at random from a Gaussian distribution with mean 10.00 and standard deviation 1.00.

Table 1.4 Simulation of a treatment where the dose of a drug is adjusted when the plasma concentration falls outside specified limits (8.50 to 11.50) even though the concentration without active adjustment would have remained in statistical control during the whole period.

Time (t)	Value without dose adjustment $X(t)$	Random change $R(t) = X(t) - X(t-1)$	Value with dose adjustment $Y(t) = Y(t-1) + R(t) + ADJ-effect(t)$ $(t > 1)$	Effect of dose adjustment ADJ-effect(t)
1	9.45		9.45	
2	7.99	−1.46	7.99	0.00
3	9.29	1.30	9.80	0.51
4	11.66	2.37	12.68	0.51
5	12.16	0.50	12.00	−1.18
6	10.18	−1.98	8.84	−1.18
7	8.04	−2.14	5.52	−1.18
8	11.46	3.42	11.92	2.98
9	9.20	−2.26	9.24	−0.42
10	10.34	1.14	9.96	−0.42
11	9.03	−1.31	8.23	−0.42
12	11.47	2.44	10.94	0.27
13	10.51	−0.96	10.25	0.27
14	9.40	−1.11	9.41	0.27
15	10.08	0.68	10.36	0.27

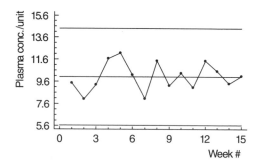

Figure 1.5 $\overline{X}$ chart, calculated from 15 random numbers generated by a Gaussian distribution with mean 10.00 and standard deviation 1.00, simulating the time course of the drug concentration measured in a patient receiving constant daily doses.

Figure 1.5 shows an $\overline{X}$ chart for $n = 1$, (see Chapter 2) constructed from these data and with the 15 values entered. As expected, the chart shows the picture one would expect when monitoring a process in statistical control the results of which follow a Gaussian distribution. The data points are all within the control limits.

Assume that the numbers represent the results of weekly measurements of the plasma concentration of a drug measured in the same patient who is taking this drug daily, without changing the dose (the basic dose). We want to calculate what would have happened if the dose, instead of having been kept constant, had been controlled by two limits, 11.50 and 8.50, as follows: when the concentration exceeds the upper limit of 11.50, the basic dose is reduced. The aim is to reduce the concentration by a quantity equal to the observed deviation from the 11.50 upper limit. In the same way, the basic dose is increased when the lower limit is exceeded.

When the dose is not adjusted, each new value is equal to the previous value plus the random biological variation that takes place between the measurements. When the dose is adjusted, the effect of the adjustment of the dose has to be added to the random biological variation. The random variation in the drug level, between measurements, is calculated as the difference between the measurements obtained when no adjustment is made. These random variations are shown in column 3 of Table 1.4. For example, the random variation from the first to the second value is $7.99 - 9.45 = -1.46$. Column 5 shows the change in the level, intended by adjustment of the basic dose according to the strategy. The values obtained when the strategy is applied and works as intended are shown in column 4. The initial value is 9.45. This is within the limits (8.50 and 11.50). So the dose is not adjusted. The second value is equal to the previous value (9.45) plus the random variation that is -1.46 and the effect of adjustment that is 0. Therefore, the second value is 7.99. This value is 0.51 below the lower limit of 8.50. Consequently, the basic dose is adjusted to increase the concentration by 0.51. So it is assumed that everything else being equal the dose adjustment increases the concentration by 0.51 until the next time where the dose is changed relative to the basic dose. The third value is equal to 7.99 plus the random variation that is 1.30, plus the effect of the adjustment of the dose that is 0.51. Therefore, the third value is 9.80. Since the value is within the limits, the current dose is not changed. The fourth value becomes equal to $9.80 + 2.37$ (the random change) $+ 0.51 = 12.68$. Now the basic dose has to be adjusted again to achieve a change of $11.50 - 12.68 = -1.18$, etc.

Calculating the mean and standard deviation of the two series, we get mean $= 10.02$ and standard deviation $= 1.28$ for the series without dose adjustment and mean $= 9.77$ and standard deviation $= 1.79$ for the series resulting from dose adjustment. Without adjustment, the mean is 0.2% away from the intended value of 10 and the standard deviation is 28% larger than 1. With active adjustment the values are 2.3% and 79% respectively. In other words, the quality of the treatment has declined considerably.

Clearly, the example is invented and rather simple-minded. However, it illustrates a phenomenon that is well known within the field of statistical process control, namely that the quality of a process that is in a state of statistical control deteriorates if one tries to adjust it on the basis of sample values. It is necessary to assess if the process is satisfactory or not, on the basis of its parameter values. If not, it must be adjusted. One then has to wait until a new state of statistical control has been reached. Then a decision has to be made if the quality of the revised process is satisfactory, etc.

1.8.2   Changing a Process That is Not in Statistical Control

RG Carey [5] reports some very interesting examples. Using somewhat modified data, but without changing the basic ideas, we present these examples. They illustrate that the interpretation of the effect of an adjustment of a process may be very difficult if the process is not in a state of statistical control.

Example 1.6

The annual death rate of coronary artery bypass graft operations at a hospital was 5 % in 1994. The protocol for the operation was changed in

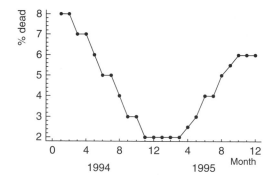

Figure 1.6   Percent of patients who died during coronary artery bypass graft operation as measured monthly during 1994 and 1995. The protocol for the operation was changed on January first 1995.

January 1995, and in January 1996 the annual death rate of 1995 was calculated and found to be 4 %. A statistical analysis comparing the annual death rates showed that this improvement was statistically significant.

Figure 1.6 shows the monthly death rates recorded during 1994 and 1995. It is obvious that for some unknown reason (perhaps improvement of the surgeons' skill to operate) the death rate has been declining throughout 1994, whereupon the trend has turned. In the beginning of 1995 the death rate dropped to 2 %, but at the end of the year it was as high as 6 %. Without examining whether the process is stable or not one may reach the conclusion that the change of protocol had a beneficial effect on the death rate. However, by examining the process, one realises that it is inappropriate to compare the annual rates because the process examined is not in a state of statistical control. In fact, inspection of the monthly rates leaves one with the impression that the change in protocol had a harmful effect.

Example 1.7

At two departments, A and B, the protocol for open-heart surgery was changed to reduce the transport time from the operating theatre to the intensive care department. The transport time is finished when the patient has stabilised and the monitoring of the patient begins. After the change in protocol had been instituted, the annual mean value of

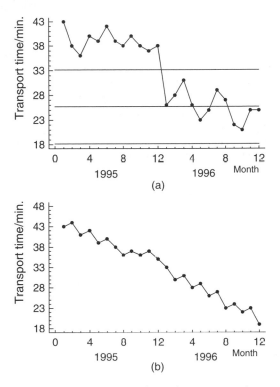

Figure 1.7 (a) The average transport time from the operating theatre to the intensive care unit as measured monthly during 1995 and 1996 in department A. The protocol for open-heart surgery was changed on January 1 1996. Only the control limits of the 1996 data are shown in the figure. (b) Data from Department B corresponding to those shown in Figure 1.7 (a) for Department A.

the transport times decreased from 39 minute to 26 minute in both departments.

Figure 1.7 (a) depicts the monthly average transport times in department A prior to and subsequent to the change in protocol. The transport time is in statistical control before as well as after the change has been introduced (only the control limits of the second period are shown in the figure). Further, the mean transport time has been reduced significantly as a result of the change. Looking at the corresponding figure for Department B, Figure 1.7 (b), one notes that the picture is completely different. Neither before nor after the introduction of the change is the process in statistical control. Furthermore, it is doubtful if the change in the protocol has had any appreciable effect on the steady decline of the monthly average transport time that started in 1995 and continued throughout 1996.

REFERENCES

[1] Shewhart WA. Quality control charts. AT&T Tech J 1926; 5:593–606.

[2] Beiles CB, Morton AP. Cumulative sum control charts for assessing performance in arterial surgery. ANZ J Surg 2004; 74:146–51.

[3] Cox DR. Planning of Experiments. John Wiley and Sons Inc, New York, 1958.

[4] Kotz S, Johnson S. Encyclopedia of Statistical Sciences 1. John Wiley and Sons Inc, New York, 1982 p351–2.

[5] Carey RG. Measuring health care quality. How do you know your care has improved? Eval Health Prof 2000; 23:43–57.

2

Shewhart Control Charts

The $\overline{X}$ chart that was mentioned in Chapter 1 is a specific example of a Shewhart chart. A formal definition of a Shewhart chart follows. Assume that samples are selected from a production process to characterise and monitor the quality of the products. Let W be a sample statistic calculated from the results obtained by measuring in each product a quantity that reflects the quality of the product (a quality indicator or measure). As long as the process is in statistical control, W follows a probability distribution with mean μ_w and standard deviation σ_w. A Shewhart control chart depicting the values of W is defined by the following equations

$$\text{UCL} = \mu_w + k\sigma_w \qquad (2.1)$$
$$\text{centreline} = \mu_w \qquad (2.2)$$
$$\text{LCL} = \mu_w - k\sigma_w \qquad (2.3)$$

where k is the distance between each control limit and the centreline measured in standard deviation. Usually $k = 3$. It is assumed that the process variables are statistically independent and that their values are generated by the same probability distribution as long as the process is in statistical control.

The sample statistics may be divided into two groups, comprising discrete and continuous sample statistics, respectively. The former are calculated by using discrete data and the latter by using continuous data. In Section 2.1 we deal with the control charts for discrete sample statistics and in Section 2.2 with control charts for continuous data.

Statistical Development of Quality in Medicine   P. Winkel and N. F. Zhang
© 2007 John Wiley & Sons, Ltd

In medical applications control charts for variable sample size may be more practical to use than control charts for equal sample size. In Section 2.3, control charts that may be used in the presence of varying sample size are expounded.

2.1 CONTROL CHARTS FOR DISCRETE DATA

Discrete data are based on a counting process. The latter may consist of counting of defective (nonconforming) and nondefective (conforming) elements in the sample. Another approach is to count the number of defects (nonconformities) per product. In the latter case the sample is viewed as a unit of products, and the result is reported as the number of defects per unit. The p control chart is used to monitor the fraction (p) of nonconforming products per sample. The c control chart is used to follow the number of nonconformities per unit of products.

2.1.1 Number of Nonconforming Products (The p Chart)

2.1.1.1 Applications

The p chart is used when products are classified as nonconforming or conforming.

The result of the inspection of a random sample of products is expressed as the number of nonconforming products found in the sample, divided by the sample size (n). An example is the inspection of patients who have undergone some operation. A 'nonconforming product' is a patient who died during the operation.

2.1.1.2 The distribution, mean value, and standard deviation of the sample statistic

Each product in a sample may be viewed as the result of an experiment. For example, a surgical procedure that has two possible outcomes: a nonconforming product (the patient dies) or a conforming one (the patient survives). We define a random variable X_i (the process variable) that may assume the values 0 or 1. $X_i = 1$ if the product is nonconforming and $X_i = 0$ if it is not. The probability that $X_i = 1$ is p, and the probability that $X_i = 0$ is $1 - p (0 < p < 1)$. D, the number of nonconforming (or defective) elements resulting from n independent experiments of this type, is a random variable defined as $D = \sum_{i=1}^{n} X_i$. As explained in appendix A, this implies that D follows a binomial distribution with parameters n and p, mean value np, and standard deviation $\sqrt{np(1-p)}$. With this assumption, it may be shown that $\frac{D}{n}$ follows a distribution with mean p and standard deviation $\sqrt{\frac{p(1-p)}{n}}$.

2.1.1.3 Estimating the mean value and standard deviation of the sample statistic

$\hat{p}$, the estimator of the parameter p, is the sum of nonconforming products found in the samples divided by the number of products inspected. We have

$$\hat{p} = \frac{\sum_{j=1}^{k} D_j}{kn} \tag{2.4}$$

where D_j is the observed number of nonconforming products in the jth sample, n the number of products per sample, and k the number of samples selected. The mean value ($\mu_{D/n}$) and standard deviation ($\sigma_{D/n}$) of p are estimated by inserting $\hat{p}$ in the equations of the mean and standard deviation. We have

$$\hat{\mu}_{D/n} = \hat{p} \tag{2.5}$$

$$\hat{\sigma}_{D/n} = \sqrt{\frac{\hat{p}(1-\hat{p})}{n}} \tag{2.6}$$

2.1.1.4 The control chart

If p is known, the p chart has

$$\text{UCL} = p + 3\sqrt{\frac{p(1-p)}{n}} \tag{2.7}$$

$$\text{centreline} = p \tag{2.8}$$

$$\text{LCL} = \max\left\{0; p - 3\sqrt{\frac{p(1-p)}{n}}\right\} \tag{2.9}$$

If p is unknown, $\hat{\mu}_{D/n}$ and $\hat{\sigma}_{D/n}$ are used in the above equations.

Example 2.1

In a clinical laboratory (many years ago) two technologists, working independently of each other, entered manually into a computer all test requests twice. Therefore, the number of errors not caught and corrected was practically 0, as had also been documented. To save manpower, the management considered purchasing an automated request form reader. The request forms were filled using a pencil to mark the tests requested. However, completing the request forms required a certain data discipline by the users. The marks had to be placed exactly as indicated on the forms, using a pencil. The laboratory borrowed the request form reader to test it out and distributed the new request forms throughout the hospital, including instructions explaining how to complete them. The testing of the request form reader lasted 20 days. Each day, all request forms were entered manually into the computer using the usual procedure, and in addition the first 300 were entered using the request form reader.

Table 2.1 shows the number (column 1) as well as the fraction (column 2) of request forms incorrectly read by the request form reader on each of the 20 days. Using Equation (2.4), $\hat{p}$ is calculated as the number of incorrectly read forms divided by the number of forms read during the trial period, i.e., $\frac{118}{6000} = 0.0197$. Using Equation (2.6), $\hat{\sigma}$ is calculated as $\sqrt{\frac{0.0197(1-0.0197)}{300}} = 0.00802$. According to Equations (2.7), (2.8), and

Table 2.1 The daily frequency and relative frequency of incorrectly read request forms per 300 forms read by an automated request form reader.

Number of incorrectly read forms	Fraction of incorrectly read forms
6	0.0200
6	0.0200
8	0.0267
7	0.0233
3	0.0100
10	0.0333
8	0.0267
2	0.0067
4	0.0133
1	0.0033
5	0.0167
8	0.0267
2	0.0067
3	0.0100
5	0.0167
2	0.0067
6	0.0200
5	0.0167
12	0.0400
15	0.0500

(2.9) the p chart of the fraction of incorrectly read request forms has:

$$\text{UCL} = 0.0197 + 3 \cdot 0.00802 = 0.0438$$
$$\text{centreline} = 0.0197$$
$$\text{LCL} = \max\{0; 0.0197 - 3 \cdot 0.00802\} = 0.$$

Here, we have used the normal approximation of the binomial distribution. If $p < \frac{1}{n+1}$ or $p > \frac{n}{n+1}$ this approximation cannot be used. Instead, the binomial distribution has to be used.

Figure 2.1 (a) shows the p chart. It appears that the process is not in control because the last sample value lies above the UCL. By reviewing the data, the management found that during the last two days of the trial a newly employed physician, using a ball pen, had filled some of the forms. In almost all of these cases the request form reader had incorrectly read the corresponding forms. Figure 2.1 (b) shows the p chart calculated

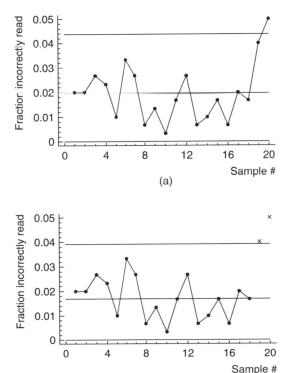

Figure 2.1 (a) p chart showing the fraction of incorrectly read request forms. (b) The revised p chart of Figure 2.1 (a). The two values excluded from the calculation of the chart are depicted as crosses.

after the last two values had been excluded. Now, the process seems to be in control with an average percentage of incorrectly read forms equal to 1.69 %. The management enjoined the clinical departments using a pencil and decided to purchase the request form reader.

2.1.2   Number of Defects (The c Chart)

Various variants of the same type of control chart may be used to monitor the number of defects (nonconformities) per unit. One of them may be used when the sample size varies (see Section 2.3.2). Here only the simplest one will be mentioned, namely the c chart.

2.1.2.1   Applications

In many instances, it is more expedient to note the number of the defects in a product than just classify it as defective or nondefective. The latter approach is simply too crude to acknowledge the variation in quality of the products. Usually the quantity reported is the number of defects per inspection unit of products. An inspection unit may consist of a single product. However, it may also include more than one product, e.g., five patients if the 'product' in question is a patient. The choice of the size of the inspection unit depends on what is practical and convenient. In some cases, the concept of a product may even be meaningless, e.g., if the defects considered are breakdowns of a hospital information system. In this case, the inspection unit is a period, e.g., a month.

2.1.2.2   The distribution, mean value, and standard deviation of the sample statistic

A Poisson distribution is often convenient to use when one is characterising the distribution of the number of defects per inspection unit because one is observing the occurrence of a random phenomenon per unit. When the Poisson distribution is applied, it is assumed that (1) the number of possible defects is infinitely large and (2) that the probability of occurrence of a defect is everywhere equally small. In practice, the mentioned conditions may only be roughly approximated. As long as the deviations from the theoretical assumptions are not significant, the Poisson distribution usually works reasonably well. The number of defects per inspection unit (DF) is assumed to follow a Poisson distribution. The Poisson distribution's parameter (here denoted c) is the mean of the distribution, and $\sqrt{c}$ is its standard deviation.

2.1.2.3 Estimating the mean value and standard deviation of the sample statistic

c is estimated as the average number of defects per inspection unit. We have:

$$\hat{c} = \frac{\sum\limits_{i=1}^{k} DF_i}{k} \qquad (2.10)$$

DF_i is the number of defects in the ith inspection unit, and k is the number of inspection units. The mean value of the sample statistic ($\mu_{DF} = c$) is estimated as:

$$\hat{\mu}_{DF} = \hat{c} \qquad (2.11)$$

and its standard deviation (σ_{DF}) is estimated as:

$$\hat{\sigma}_{DF} = \sqrt{\hat{c}} \qquad (2.12)$$

2.1.2.4 The control chart

c is the mean value of the sample statistic, and $\sqrt{c}$ is its standard deviation. Therefore, if c is known, the control chart has:

$$UCL = c + 3\sqrt{c} \qquad (2.13)$$
$$centreline = c \qquad (2.14)$$
$$LCL = \max\{0; c - 3\sqrt{c}\} \qquad (2.15)$$

If c is not known, the estimate of c is substituted for c in the above equations. Since the Poisson distribution is skewed to the right, especially if c is small, it is sometimes preferred to use probability limits. They are calculated by cutting off 0.135 % of the area of the distribution at each of its ends [1].

Example 2.2

The Glasgow Royal Infirmary is a tertiary referral centre that provides regional services for cardiac, burn, and bone marrow transplant patients. Table 2.2, column 1 shows the monthly count of Methicillin resistant *Staphylococcus aureus* (MRSA) cases from January 1997 through May 1998. The data are historical and originate from a study by Curran *et al.* [2]. We will calculate a c control chart using these data. c is estimated as

$$\hat{c} = \frac{25 + 34 + 19 + \ldots + 20}{17} = 29.3 \, \text{MRSA/month.}$$

Table 2.2 The monthly total acquisition of Methicillin resistant *Staphylococcus aureus* from January 1997 to May 1998 (column 1) and from June 1998 through September 2000 (column 2 and 3) in a tertiary referral centre.

January 1997 to May 1998	June 1998 to September 2000	
25	51	50
34	46	50
19	49	49
24	41	49
32	38	42
39	43	38
25	29	34
24	31	28
23	40	25
33	28	25
29	42	22
24	42	
32	44	
38	41	
39	44	
38	25	
20	54	

The c chart is calculated as

$$\text{UCL} = \hat{c} + 3\sqrt{\hat{c}} = 29.3 + 3 \cdot 5.41 = 45.5 \, \text{MRSA/month}$$

$$\text{centreline} = \hat{c} = 29.3 \, \text{MRSA/month}$$

$$\text{LCL} = \max\{0; \hat{c} - 3\sqrt{\hat{c}}\} = 13.1 \, \text{MRSA/month}.$$

Figure 2.2 (a) shows the chart with the 17 counts used to calculate it. The count is assumed to be in statistical control because none of the points are located outside the control limits. The counts recorded from June 1998 through September 2000 are shown in columns 2 and 3 in Table 2.2. Figure 2.2 (b) shows these counts depicted on the chart calculated above. From June 1998 until February 2000, eight values were higher than the UCL, and all but three values were higher than the centreline. Therefore, the rate of MRSA cases was significantly elevated during this period as compared to the previous 17 months.

From December 1999 each of the 24 wards and units in the centre received an annotated control chart based on the historical data generated

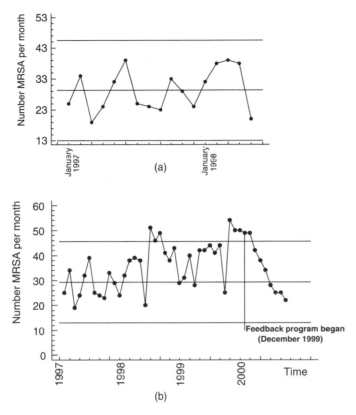

Figure 2.2 (a) *c* chart showing number of Methicillin resistant *Staphylococcus aureus* (MRSA) infections per month at a tertiary referral centre. (b) *c* chart showing number of Methicillin resistant *Staphylococcus aureus* (MRSA) infections per month at a tertiary referral centre. The first 17 values were used to calculate the *c* chart. In December 1999 a feed back program was initiated.

by that ward/unit. Results were fed back on a regular monthly basis to medical staff, ward managers, senior managers, and hotel services. If a value fell outside the control limits or prolonged runs above or below the centreline were seen the cause was investigated. If the rate had increased it was determined whether it was due to inconsistently followed infection control practices, changes in the case-mix severity or some other reason. The overall effect of this program is apparent from an inspection of Figure 2.2 (b). Two months after the feedback program had begun, monthly reductions in the acquisition rate of MRSA occurred. After that the rate remained stable at approximately 50 % of the rate before the intervention and only one medical specialty area had an out-of-control episode.

2.2 CONTROL CHARTS FOR CONTINUOUS DATA

Continuous data include the measurements of one or more properties of each element in a sample, e.g., a patient's length of stay at a hospital. If a process is in control, the values of the process variable follow a probability distribution. This may be characterised by its mean value and standard deviation. If the type of distribution and its parameters are known, the state of the process is completely described. Usually, it is assumed that the type of distribution is Gaussian. Since the two parameters (mean and standard deviation) in a Gaussian distribution are necessary and sufficient to characterise the distribution, it is recommended [1] to use two control charts to characterise the process, one chart that is used to monitor the stability of the mean and one chart that is used to monitor the stability of the standard deviation. In some situations, it is expedient to use samples comprising only one product. This creates special problems. Therefore, this situation will be dealt with separately.

2.2.1 Sample Size Larger Than 1

If the sample size is larger than 1, an $\overline{X}$ chart is used to monitor the mean of the process variable. An S chart is used to monitor the standard deviation. It is common practice to combine an $\overline{X}$ chart with an S chart. If the process standard deviation changes while the mean is stable, a marked change may be identified using the $\overline{X}$ chart. However, the S chart is much more sensitive to a change in the process standard deviation.

2.2.1.1 The S chart

The standard deviation of the measurements obtained from a sample is calculated as

$$S = \sqrt{\frac{\sum_{i=1}^{n} (X_i - \overline{X})^2}{n - 1}} \qquad (2.16)$$

where n is the sample size, X_i the ith measurement, and $\overline{X}$ the average of the measurements. A control chart using this sample statistic is referred to as an S chart.

Application The S chart is used to follow the standard deviation of the process variable.

The mean value and standard deviation of the sample statistic It may be shown that the mean value μ_S of S is

$$\mu_S = c_4\sigma \qquad (2.17)$$

where σ is the standard deviation of the process variable. The standard deviation (σ_S) of S is

$$\sigma_S = \sigma\sqrt{1 - c_4^2} \qquad (2.18)$$

The value of c_4 depends on n and may be found in Table 1.1.

Estimating the mean value and standard deviation of the sample statistic From Equation (2.17), the standard deviation (σ) of the process variable is estimated by the average of the sample standard deviations divided by c_4 that may be found in Table 1.1. c_4 adjusts for bias based on Equation (2.17). Therefore, an unbiased estimate is calculated as

$$\hat{\sigma} = \frac{\overline{S}}{c_4} \qquad (2.19)$$

where $\overline{S} - \dfrac{\sum\limits_{i=1}^{k} S_i}{k}$, k is the number of samples, and S_i the standard deviation of the ith test sample. The estimates of the mean, μ_S, and standard deviation, σ_S, of S are obtained by inserting $\frac{\overline{S}}{c_4}$ for σ in the Equations (2.17) and (2.18). We obtain

$$\hat{\mu}_S = \overline{S} \qquad (2.20)$$

and

$$\hat{\sigma}_S = \frac{\overline{S}\sqrt{1 - c_4^2}}{c_4} \qquad (2.21)$$

The control chart If σ is known, the S chart is calculated using the Equations (2.17) and (2.18). The control chart has

$$UCL = c_4\sigma + 3\sigma\sqrt{1 - c_4^2} = B_6\sigma \qquad (2.22)$$

$$centreline = c_4\sigma \qquad (2.23)$$

$$LCL = \max\{0; c_4\sigma - 3\sigma\sqrt{1 - c_4^2}\} = B_5\sigma \qquad (2.24)$$

where $B_6 = c_4 + 3\sqrt{1 - c_4^2}$, and $B_5 = \max\{0; c_4 - 3\sqrt{1 - c_4^2}\}$. The values of B_6 and B_5 depend on the sample size; they may be found in Table 1.1. If μ_S and σ_S are not known, their estimates (Equations (2.20) and (2.21)) are inserted in the above equations, and we get

$$\text{UCL} = \bar{S} + \frac{3\bar{S}\sqrt{1 - c_4^2}}{c_4} = B_4\bar{S} \qquad (2.25)$$

$$\text{centreline} = \bar{S} \qquad (2.26)$$

$$\text{LCL} = \max\left\{ 0; \left[1 - \frac{3\sqrt{1 - c_4^2}}{c_4} \right]\bar{S} \right\} = B_3\bar{S} \qquad (2.27)$$

where $B_4 = 1 + \frac{3\sqrt{1-c_4^2}}{c_4}$, and $B_3 = \max\{0; 1 - \frac{3\sqrt{1-c_4^2}}{c_4}\}$. Both quantities depend on the sample size and may be found in Table 1.1. The Equations (2.25), (2.26), and (2.27) should be used when the standard deviation of the process variable is unknown.

Example 2.3

At a clinic receiving adult outpatients the management wanted to assess the variability of the blood pressure (BP) measurements made. During 12 weekdays one patient per day was selected at random, and his/her blood pressure measured three times. The result of the first measurement was discarded because previous experiments had shown that the result of the first measurement was systematically higher than those of the two subsequent measurements.

Table 2.3 shows the results of the last two systolic and two diastolic BP measurements of each patient. The corresponding standard deviations have been calculated and are also shown in the table. We may construct an S chart using the standard deviations of the systolic blood pressure measurements. $\bar{S}$ is 4.24 mm Hg. Since σ is not known, Equations (2.25), (2.26), and (2.27) are used when the S chart is calculated. Because $n = 2$, B_3 and B_4 are equal to 0 and 3.267, respectively (see Table 1.1). Therefore, the S chart has

$$\text{UCL} = 3.267 \cdot 4.24 = 13.9\,\text{mm Hg}$$
$$\text{centreline} = 4.2\,\text{mm Hg}$$
$$\text{LCL} = 0.0\,\text{mm Hg}.$$

Table 2.3 Two measurements of the systolic and the diastolic blood pressure (BP) made in each of 12 patients.

Second systolic BP	Third systolic BP	Standard deviation of systolic BP	Second diastolic BP	Third diastolic BP	Standard deviation of diastolic BP
132	132	0.000	90	92	1.414
128	130	1.414	92	88	2.828
120	122	1.414	72	62	7.071
104	108	2.828	86	82	2.828
100	98	1.414	70	60	7.071
102	120	12.728	84	76	5.657
106	102	2.828	64	58	4.243
132	124	5.657	84	84	0.000
142	144	1.414	78	86	5.657
130	142	8.485	94	100	4.243
130	112	12.728	82	82	0.000
112	112	0.000	78	76	1.414

$\bar{S}$ of the diastolic pressures is 3.54 mm Hg. Therefore, the corresponding S chart has

$$\text{UCL} = 3.267 \cdot 3.54 = 11.6 \, \text{mm Hg}$$
$$\text{centreline} = 3.5 \, \text{mm Hg}$$
$$\text{LCL} = 0.0 \, \text{mm Hg}.$$

The two S charts are shown in Figures 2.3 (a) and 2.3 (b). On both charts the standard deviation seems to be in statistical control because all standard deviations lie below the UCL.

Subsequently, three systolic and three diastolic BPs were routinely measured in each outpatient visiting the clinic. The standard deviation of the last two measurements of each set of results was calculated and each compared to the UCL of the corresponding control chart. If it was below the UCL, the corresponding mean value was reported, and if not, a search for the cause of the excessive variation was initiated, according to a written protocol.

The data used in this example is an extract of those examined in the paper by Nelson et al. [3] (see Table 1 in the paper).

2.2.1.2 The $\bar{X}$ chart

This chart was used for illustrative purposes in Chapter 1.

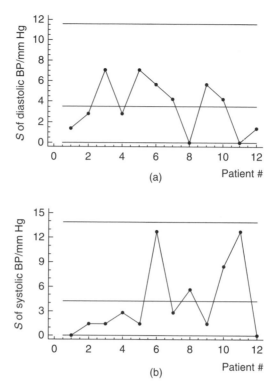

(a)   Patient #

(b)   Patient #

Figure 2.3 (a) S chart of the standard deviation (s) of two repeated measurements of the diastolic blood pressure (BP)/mm Hg made in the same patient. (b) S chart of the standard deviation (s) of two repeated measurements of the systolic blood pressure (BP)/mm Hg made in the same patient.

2.2.1.3   Interpretation of the $\overline{X}$ chart and the S chart

If a sample value falls outside the control limits, one may assume that the process is not in control. Therefore, the cause should be tracked systematically. Inspection of the control chart may help the investigation.

Figure 2.4 shows how the distribution of the sample mean values depicted on an $\overline{X}$ chart will change when the mean of the process variable changes (Figure 2.4 (a)) and when its standard deviation changes (Figure 2.4 (b)). A change of the process mean causes the values to be distributed asymmetrically, relative to the centreline. When the mean increases, the values accumulate above the centreline, and when it decreases, they accumulate below this line. The probability that a value may fall above the UCL, or below the LCL, increases. If only the standard deviation increases, the sample values will still be distributed symmetrically around the centreline. However, a larger fraction will fall

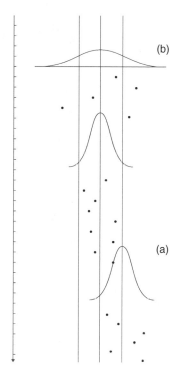

Figure 2.4 The behaviour of the $\overline{X}$ chart in the presence of various types of lack of statistical control. Frame (a) shows the pattern resulting from an increase of the process mean value. Frame (b) shows the pattern resulting from an increase of the process standard deviation.

outside the control limits. These facts may be useful to keep in mind when tracking down why a value falls outside the control limits. If a value falls outside the control limits of the $\overline{X}$ chart, one should first inspect the corresponding S chart to make sure that the standard deviation of the process variable is stable. If this is not so, the standard deviation should first be brought under control. Then, the process should be monitored using the $\overline{X}$ chart. If values still fall outside the control limits, it implies that the process mean has also changed.

When a process gets out of statistical control, the arising systematic patterns of sample values may provide valuable information about the cause of the loss of control.

Figure 2.5 shows various types of data patterns. The pattern depicted in Figure 2.5 (a) is cyclical. This type of pattern may be caused by changes in the surroundings, e.g., operator shifts, etc. The pattern shown in Figure 2.5 (b) is called 'mixed pattern'. Alternately, the values accumulate close to the UCL and close to the LCL, while few values are

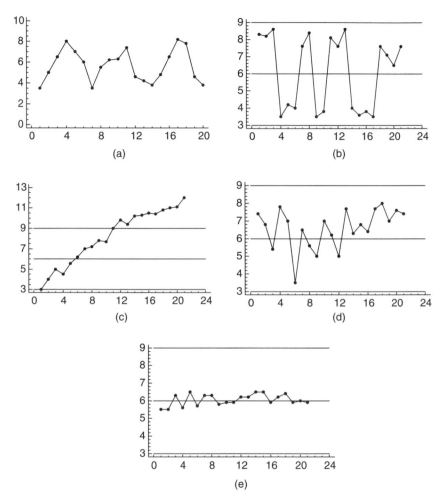

Figure 2.5 (a)–(e) Various characteristic control chart value patterns of diagnostic significance. The abscissa is the sample number, and the ordinate is the sample mean value. Since only the patterns are of interest, the x- and the y-axis are without legends (a) A cyclical pattern. (b) A mixed pattern. (c)A trend. (d)A changing level. (e) Too small a variation relative to the control limits.

located close to the centreline. This pattern may appear, e.g., when the process is excessively controlled because the operator adjusts it as a response to random variations (see Example 1.6). A trend, depicted in Figure 2.5 (c), is a continuous change of the mean in the same direction. For instance this may be seen if a problem gets increasingly serious as time goes by. Figure 2.5 (d) shows the pattern resulting from a shift in the mean of the process variable. Figure 2.5 (e) depicts a pattern of values scattered around and close to the centreline, showing little natural variation. The reason may simply be that the control limits used are set too far apart. It is also possible that for some reason the standard deviation of the process variable has decreased since the control chart was constructed.

Example 2.4

At an emergency department the management decided to monitor patient satisfaction. On each weekday during the day shift, six patients were selected at random. The physicians, treating the patients, were not aware who were the patients selected. Each of the patients received a questionnaire pertaining to his/her satisfaction with the treatment he/she had just received. From the answers, a score was calculated that theoretically ranged from 0 to 100. Table 2.4 shows the daily mean and standard deviation of the satisfaction score measured during three weeks.

The grand mean and the average of the standard deviations are also shown. The process standard deviation is estimated by $\frac{\bar{S}}{c_4} = \frac{9.64}{0.9515} = 10.13$ where c_4 may be found in Table 1.1 for $n = 6$.

We will calculate an $\overline{X}$ chart and an S chart using these data. The sample standard deviation is $\frac{10.13}{\sqrt{6}} = 4.14$ because the sample size is 6.

Table 2.4 Mean and standard deviation of satisfaction scores given by six randomly selected patients on each of 15 days.

Day #	Sample size	Mean	Standard deviation
1	6	65.96	5.95
2	6	60.27	8.98
3	6	60.80	6.65
4	6	66.40	9.54
5	6	65.39	10.34
6	6	49.18	12.13
7	6	50.38	15.15
8	6	53.71	14.98
9	6	55.46	19.26
10	6	49.20	11.09
11	6	73.58	5.94
12	6	75.25	8.18
13	6	73.17	5.99
14	6	70.72	6.88
15	6	70.47	3.50
Average		62.7	9.64

The centreline of the $\overline{X}$ chart is equal to the grand mean 62.7, and the control limits are $62.7 \pm 3 \cdot 4.14 = 50.3$ to 75.1. The centreline of the S chart is at $\overline{S} = 9.64$, the upper control limit is $9.64 \cdot B_4 = 9.64 \cdot 1.97 = 19.00$, and the lower control limit is $9.64 \cdot B_3 = 9.64 \cdot 0.030 = 0.29$, where B_4 and B_3 may be found in Table 1.1 for $n = 6$.

Figures 2.6 (a) and 2.6 (b) show the $\overline{X}$ chart and the S chart, respectively. Neither the standard deviation nor the mean is in statistical control. The $\overline{X}$ chart displays a clear cyclical pattern, with two values being outside the control limits. The S of sample # 9 lies above the upper control limit of the S chart. Usually, one should begin by examining why the standard deviation is out of control. Once the standard deviation is brought under control, one may proceed to see if the mean is still out of control. But in this case, the cycles of the $\overline{X}$ chart give us a clue. The shifts

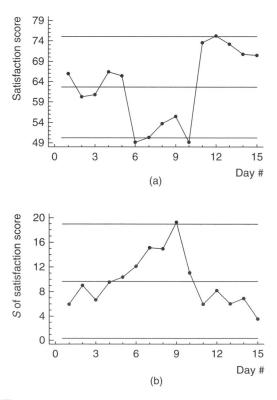

(a)

(b)

Figure 2.6 (a) $\overline{X}$ chart depicting the mean value of the satisfaction score measured in six patients randomly selected on each of 15 consecutive weekdays. (b) S chart depicting the standard deviation (S) of the satisfaction score measured in six patients randomly selected on each of 15 consecutive weekdays.

Table 2.5 Schedule showing when each of six physicians attended the emergency department during three consecutive weeks.

Week #	1	2	3
Physicians attending	# 1 # 2	# 3 # 4	# 5 # 6

between the cycles coincide in time with the shifts between weeks. Therefore, we should look for anything that varied systematically from week to week during the three-week period.

Table 2.5 shows the day shift calendar for the 15 days. It is noted that physicians # 1 and # 2 shared the daily shift during the first week. Then physician # 3 and # 4 took over, and during the last week physicians # 5 and # 6 shared the daily shift. Therefore, a likely explanation of the findings is that the physicians differ in terms of the satisfaction scores they received.

Figure 2.7 shows a Boxplot of the satisfaction scores received by each of the six physicians. A statistical test (a one way analysis of variance comparing the six mean values) supported the impression given by this figure, namely that the mean of the received satisfaction scores differed significantly among the physicians. Physician specific control charts (not shown) revealed that the satisfaction score of each physician was in statistical control. Based on this analysis, physician specific control charts were used from then on.

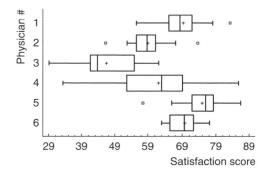

Figure 2.7 Boxplot of the satisfaction scores received by each of six physicians. Each box represents the values of one physician. Fifty percent of the scores have values within the box that is delimited by the 25th and 75th percentiles. Inside the box the mean (the cross) and the median (vertical line) are depicted. The lines are drawn from the end of the box to the smallest observation (left line) and the largest observation (right line) that is not an outlier. The small boxes at the same level as the large box depict the remaining, outlying scores received by the physician.

2.2.2 Individual Observations

Under certain circumstances, it may be more expedient to use a sample comprising just one product. This may be required if the process is very slow or the variation within a test sample is unrealistically small as compared to the variation one wants to control. The standard deviation of the process variable cannot be estimated based on a sample comprising only one product. However, constructing a sample comprising two consecutively sampled products when estimating the standard deviation may solve this problem. The two samples are considered as one sample in this context. Then, one uses the range of the sample when calculating an estimate of the process standard deviation. Two consecutive ranges share one value (the middle one). A range calculated in this way is called a moving range (MR_i).

Example 2.5

The following data set consists of six sample values: $\{1, 4, 2, 7, 2, 4\}$. The corresponding five values of the MR_i are calculated as follows:
$MR_1 = 4-1=3; \quad MR_2 = 4-2=2; \quad MR_3 = 7-2=5; \quad MR_4 = 7-2=5;$
$MR_5 = 4 - 2 = 2.$
$\overline{MR}$, the mean of the moving ranges is $\frac{3+2+5+5+2}{5} = 3.4$.

2.2.2.1 The X chart

The control chart for single observations is referred to as an X chart.

Application This chart is used to monitor the mean of the process variable.

The distribution, the mean value, and the standard deviation of the sample statistic Each sample consists of one product. X is assumed to follow a Gaussian distribution with mean μ and standard deviation σ.

Estimating the distribution, mean value, and standard deviation of the sample statistic The mean value (μ) of the sample statistic is estimated as

$$\overline{X} = \frac{\sum_{i=1}^{k} X_i}{k} \tag{2.28}$$

where X_i is the random variable corresponding to the ith sample value and k the number of samples. σ can be estimated by

$$\hat{\sigma}_{\text{MR}} = \frac{\sum\limits_{j=2}^{k} |X_j - X_{j-1}|}{d_2(k-1)} = \frac{\overline{\text{MR}}}{1.128} \qquad (2.29)$$

where $|X_j - X_{j-1}|$ is the $(j-1)$th MR, and d_2 is a constant equal to 1.128.

The control chart If μ and σ are known the X chart has

$$\text{UCL} = \mu + 3\sigma \qquad (2.30)$$
$$\text{centreline} = \mu \qquad (2.31)$$
$$\text{LCL} = \mu - 3\sigma \qquad (2.32)$$

If μ and σ are not known, the X chart has

$$\text{UCL} = \overline{X} + 3\frac{\overline{\text{MR}}}{1.128} \qquad (2.33)$$
$$\text{centreline} = \overline{X} \qquad (2.34)$$
$$\text{LCL} = \overline{X} - 3\frac{\overline{\text{MR}}}{1.128} \qquad (2.35)$$

where $\overline{X}$ is the mean of the random variables corresponding to the samples examined. A chart corresponding to the S chart may be calculated (a MR chart). However, it is not particularly useful since it will react to changes in the mean value as well as changes in the standard deviation. Therefore, usually, only the X chart is used in the presence of single observations.

Example 2.6

The risk of infection is usually estimated by the relative frequency of infections, i.e., the number of patients who have acquired an infection during a specified period divided by the number of patients who have been exposed to the risk of getting an infection during that period. When one is monitoring the relative frequency of infections, rather large patient samples are usually required to ensure that each patient sample contains a few infected patients. This implies that the main significance of the samples is only a matter of history since it will usually be too late to take any action when a sufficiently large sample of patients has finally been collected. Therefore, recording the period between consecutive infections is often used instead. If the number of patients exposed to the risk of being infected is constant over time, the period between infections will decrease as the relative frequency of infections increases, and vice versa.

The data used in the present example were read from a figure in a study by Finison et al [4]. In this study, the relation between the number of days elapsed between consecutively registered *Clostridium difficile* infections and the sequence number of the infections was examined using an X chart, depicting the former versus the latter and calculated using the first six values. The authors found that the distribution of the periods is highly skewed to the right. The data are better described using an exponential probability distribution. Therefore, one approach is to construct a control chart, based on this type of distribution [5]. Alternatively, one may transform the data and then depict the transformed values, using the conventional X chart. To arrive at a Gaussian distribution from an exponential one, it is recommended [6] to use the transformation $Y = X^{0.2777}$ where X is the original variable and Y the transformed one. We will use this approach.

Table 2.6 shows the sequential number of each infection (column 1) and the number of days elapsed between this and the subsequent infection (column 2). The corresponding value obtained using the above transformation is also shown (column 3).

Figure 2.8 shows an X chart depicting the transformed value versus the infection #, calculated using the first six transformed values; these and the subsequent 18 values have been entered on the chart. The period between the 11th and the 12th infection exceeds the UCL. The most likely explanation is that the laboratory had some problems with the *Clostridium difficile* assay so that the presence of *Clostridium difficile* was sometimes overlooked. None of the values lie below the LCL. However, one suspects that the process has changed since the last 11 values are located below the inner lower warning limit. The X chart may profitably be combined with an exponentially weighted moving average (EWMA) chart. Therefore, we will continue this example in Chapter 3 where we examine the EWMA chart. Usually one would use more than six values to calculate the chart. However, to be able to start the monitoring without too much delay it may be practical initially to use fewer values than usual.

Table 2.6 The number of days between registered *Clostridium difficile* infections.

Infection #	Number of days elapsed between present and subsequent infection (x)	$x^{0.2777}$ (y)
1	30	2.572
2	18	2.231
3	31	2.595
4	129	3.856
5	102	3.612
6	18	2.231
7	8	1.782
8	6	1.645
9	19	2.265
10	169	4.156
11	283	4.796
12	99	3.583
13	75	3.317
14	4	1.470
15	3	1.357
16	2	1.212
17	3	1.357
18	4	1.470
19	5	1.564
20	1	1.000
21	1	1.000
22	14	2.081
23	8	1.782
24	9	1.841

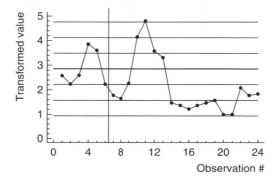

Figure 2.8 X chart showing the transformed value of number of days in between consecutive registered cases of *Clostridium difficile* infections. Control limits and upper and lower warning limits, three, two, and one standard deviations removed from the centreline, respectively, are depicted on the chart. The chart was constructed using the first 6 values.

Example 2.7

A patient suffering from asthma made daily measurements of her peak
expiratory flow rate (PEFR) in the morning, prior to bronchodilator
treatment. The results of the first 19 measurements (see Table 2.7)
were used to calculate an X chart. If the values of the X chart are all
within the control limits, the patient's PEFR is stable. This is only a good
thing if the patient is stable at a level that is clinically acceptable. Special
causes may disturb a given balance, no matter whether the latter is
clinically satisfying or not, and cause additional variation. These causes
may be a sudden change in the patient's exposure to allergens, a change
in unspecific irritation, or the appearance of infections.

Figure 2.9 (a) shows the X chart, calculated using the 19 values that
are also depicted on the chart. Value # 13 lies above the UCL, and 3 out
of 4 consecutive values (# 10, # 11, # 12, and # 13) lie above the outer
upper warning limit (294 l/min) not shown. Therefore, the patient's state
is not stable. As it turned out, during the period when the four values had
been measured the patient had lived with her aunt. Here the patient was
no longer exposed to a dog, tobacco smoke, or mites. Therefore, the
values # 10, # 11, # 12, and # 13 were deleted, and a revised control chart

Table 2.7 Peak expiratory flow rate/l/minute (PEFR) measured daily in
the morning in the same patient suffering from asthma.

Day #	PEFR before change of treatment	Day #	PEFR after change of treatment
1	121	1	310
2	140	2	307
3	99	3	325
4	150	4	346
5	268	5	380
6	150	6	312
7	100	7	384
8	122	8	376
9	152	9	354
10	315	10	370
11	321	11	365
12	275	12	325
13	367	13	368
14	200	14	350
15	138		
16	175		
17	150		
18	150		
19	180		

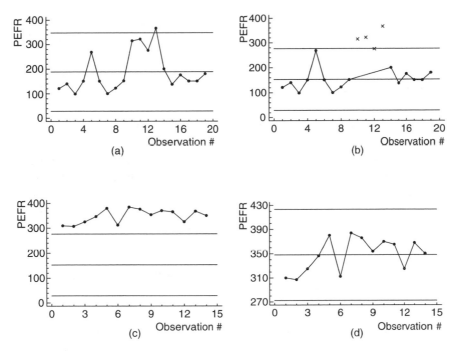

Figure 2.9 (a) X chart showing the peak expiratory flow rate/l/minute (PEFR) measured daily in the same patient suffering from asthma. (b) X chart showing peak expiratory flow rate/l/minute (PEFR) measured daily in the same patient. The chart was calculated using the values shown in Figure 2.9 (a), following exclusion of values # 10, # 11, # 12, and # 13, depicted as crosses. (c) X chart showing peak expiratory flow rate/l/minute (PEFR) measured daily in the same patient. The X chart was calculated using values measured in the same patient, prior to a change in therapy (see Figure 2.9 (b)). The 14 PEFR values depicted on the X chart were measured after the treatment had been changed and starting two weeks after the change had been initiated. (d) X chart calculated from the peak expiratory flow rate/l/minute (PEFR) values depicted in Figure 2.9 (c). These values are shown on the X chart.

was calculated, using the remaining values. The purpose of this was to see if the patient's condition was stable when she was staying at her home, and if so, to learn what the nature of her condition would then be. The mean value of the remaining 15 values was 153.00 l/min, and $\overline{MR}$ was 46.50 l/min. Using these results, the estimate of the process standard deviation is calculated to be $\hat{\sigma} = \frac{46.50}{1.128} = 41.22$ l/min. The X chart has UCL $= 153.00 + 3 \cdot 41.22 = 276.66$ l/min, centreline $= 153.00$ l/min, and LCL $= 153.00 - 3 \cdot 41.22 = 29.34$ l/min.

Figure 2.9 (b) shows the X chart with the values entered. Now, the patient's condition appears to be stable. However, it is clinically unsatisfactory since a few negative external influences may cause the patient to develop an asthma attack. Therefore, the treatment schedule was altered, taking advantage of the experiences gained from the patient's stay at her aunt's house. Figure 2.9 (c) shows 14 daily values measured after the patient had been subjected to the new treatment for some time. The values have been entered on the original X chart shown in Figure 2.9 (b). Since all values lie above the UCL, it is quite clear that the change of treatment (changing the system) has brought the patient out of her previous stable, but clinically unsatisfying, condition. The question, now, is if the patient's new condition is stable. Figure 2.9 (d) shows the X chart, calculated using the last 14 values that are depicted on the chart. Since they all lie within the control limits, it appears that the patient's new and improved condition is stable. The data used in this example have been extracted from a paper by Boggs *et al.* [7] and modified slightly.

2.3 CONTROL CHARTS FOR VARIABLE SAMPLE SIZE

When control charts are used for clinical purposes, each sample often includes all patients seen during a specified period, e.g., a month. This implies that the sample size may vary. However, it is often more convenient and practical to use equally sized sampling periods instead of equally sized samples when sampling the entire production. Among the control charts presented so far, the p chart and the combination $\overline{X}$ chart and S chart may be used when the sample size is varying.

2.3.1 The p Chart

The centreline of the p chart with varying sample size is the same as that of the chart with equal sample size. However, the control limits are different. We have

$$UCL_i = p + 3\sqrt{\frac{p(1-p)}{n_i}} \qquad (2.36)$$

and

$$LCL_i = \max\left\{0; p - 3\sqrt{\frac{p(1-p)}{n_i}}\right\} \qquad (2.37)$$

where n_i is the size of the ith sample. If p is unknown, $\hat{p}$ is calculated as

$$\hat{p} = \frac{\sum\limits_{i=1}^{k} D_i}{\sum\limits_{i=1}^{k} n_i} \qquad (2.38)$$

where k is the number of samples, D_i the number of nonconforming products in the ith test sample, and n_i its size. When p is unknown, p is replaced by $\hat{p}$ in Equations (2.36) and (2.37).

Example 2.8

Anaesthetic mortality and serious morbidity occur infrequently and, therefore, have limited value as indicators of quality of the anaesthetic process in a single institution. However, less serious intraoperative adverse events may change the patient's postoperative course and are associated with the development of 'critical' events. Therefore, they may be observed to monitor the safety and quality of the anaesthetic process. At the Trondheim University Hospital [8], Fasting and Gisvold examined the frequency of recorded adverse events in data retrieved from the department database from 1997 to 2001. We present the results of their analysis of the occurrence of difficult emergence from general anaesthesia that may be associated with life threatening problems with the airways or circulation during awakening. The results were reconstructed from a reading of their figures. Patients younger than 16 years of age and/or having cardiac anaesthesia were excluded. During the period 1997 to 2001, 1123 difficult emergences from general anaesthesia occurred out of a total of 45 088 general anaesthesias, giving an average ($\hat{p}$) of 0.025.

Table 2.8 shows the number of difficult emergences, the number of anaesthesias given, and the fraction of difficult emergence for each bimonthly period for a total of 30 periods during the five-year period from 1997 to 2001.

Figure 2.10 (a) shows the p chart calculated, using all data. The process is not in control. Two values are outside the control limits, and 14 out of the last 16 values lie below the centreline. It turned out that during the first quarter of 1999 the occurrence of difficult emergence had been deemed unacceptably high. It had been found out that, in all

Table 2.8 The number of general anaesthesias given, the number of difficult emergences from anaesthesia, and the rate of difficult emergence from anaesthesia during each of 30 bimonthly periods. After period # 14 a preventive program (intervention) was initiated.

Bimonthly period #	Number of general anaesthesias from anaesthesia	Number of difficult emergences anaesthesia	Rate of difficult emergence from
1	1489	45	0.030
2	1466	45	0.031
3	1527	47	0.031
4	1579	55	0.035
5	1451	43	0.030
6	1567	36	0.023
7	1446	44	0.030
8	1520	41	0.027
9	1526	49	0.032
10	1452	54	0.037
11	1454	33	0.023
12	1436	46	0.032
13	1457	47	0.032
14	1562	47	0.030
Intervention			
15	1484	22	0.015
16	1458	31	0.021
17	1535	26	0.017
18	1547	28	0.018
19	1482	22	0.015
20	1579	38	0.024
21	1463	32	0.022
22	1529	29	0.019
23	1452	31	0.021
24	1480	38	0.026
25	1519	17	0.011
26	1458	36	0.025
27	1570	36	0.023
28	1534	29	0.019
29	1560	41	0.026
30	1506	35	0.023

likelihood, the problems were due to residual drug effect or misjudgement of the patient's respiratory status before extubation. Therefore, as part of a preventive program initiated, long-acting muscular relaxants had been replaced by intermediate-acting muscular relaxants. During the first 14 bimonthly periods (1997, 1998 and the first two months of 1999), there were 632 difficult emergences out of 20 932 anaesthesias given. This gives a $\hat{p}$ value of $\frac{632}{20.932} = 0.030$. Figure 2.10 (b) shows the

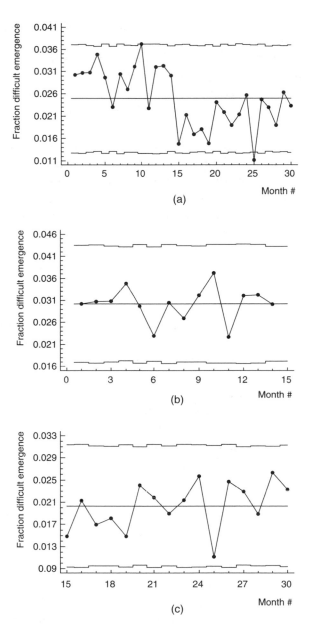

Figure 2.10 (a) p chart for variable sample size showing the fraction of difficult emergence from anaesthesia recorded during each of 30 bimonthly periods. All data depicted were used to calculate the chart. The process is not in statistical control. (b) p chart for variable sample size showing fraction of difficult emergence from anaesthesia recorded during each of the first 14 bimonthly periods depicted in Figure 2.10 (a). The data from all 14 periods were used to calculate the chart. The process is in statistical control. (c) A p chart for variable sample size showing fraction of difficult emergence from anaesthesia recorded during each of the last 16 bimonthly periods depicted in Figure 2.10 (a). The data from all 16 periods were used to calculate the chart. The process is in statistical control.

control chart obtained using this value as the centreline. The first 14 fraction values with corresponding control limits are also depicted in the figure. It shows the picture of a process in control. During the last 16 bimonthly periods, there were 491 difficult emergences out of 24 156 anaesthesias given. This gives an average value of $\frac{491}{24\,156} = 0.020$. Figure 2.10 (c) shows the control chart based on this value. It depicts the last 16 values and corresponding control limits. This also is the picture of a process in control. However, now the process has stabilised at a significantly lower mean fraction of difficult emergence (0.020 which is significantly lower than 0.030). It appears that changing the system improved the quality.

Example 2.9

In a study by Norberg et al [9] conducted at a children's hospital emergency department, it was hypothesised that the blood culture contamination rate would be less when blood culture specimens were obtained from a remote site, rather than through a newly inserted intravenous catheter. To test this hypothesis, blood specimens for culture were first obtained simultaneously with intravenous catheter insertion during a baseline phase (January 1, 1998 to November 19, 1998). These data served as baseline data. During a six-week implementation phase (November 20, 1998 – December 31, 1998), the specimens were obtained by a separate, dedicated procedure. This specimen collection procedure was then continued during the post intervention phase (January 1, 1999 – December 31, 1999). The infectious disease expert was without knowledge of the intervention phase, and the nursing staff members were unaware of the ongoing data collection and analysis.

Table 2.9 shows the data. During the baseline period of 10 months, 2113 culture specimens were collected; 191 were contaminated. $\hat{p}$, the mean fraction contaminated during this phase, was $\frac{191}{2113} = 0.090$. Using this level, the control limits of each of the 22 months may be calculated by inserting $\hat{p}$ and the number of specimens collected during the month in Equations (2.36) and (2.37). For example, for month # 1 we obtain the limits: $0.090 \pm 3\sqrt{\frac{0.090(1-0.090)}{212}} = 0.090 \pm 0.059 = 0.031$ to 0.150. The observed fraction of this month (0.099) lies within the control limits.

Figure 2.11 (a) shows the p chart constructed, using the mean rate obtained from the data collected during the initial 10 months. The

Table 2.9 Number of blood cultures obtained, number contaminated, and fraction of contaminated blood cultures on each of 22 consecutive months. Results obtained during the first 10 months served as baseline data. Subsequently blood culture specimens were obtained from a remote site (intervention).

Month #	Number of blood cultures obtained	Number of contaminated cultures	Fraction of contaminated cultures
1	212	21	0.099
2	212	22	0.104
3	211	14	0.066
4	211	12	0.057
5	214	26	0.122
6	212	15	0.071
7	208	20	0.096
8	214	17	0.079
9	208	16	0.077
10	211	28	0.133
Intervention			
11	169	4	0.024
12	165	2	0.012
13	169	6	0.036
14	168	2	0.012
15	168	8	0.048
16	169	8	0.047
17	171	5	0.029
18	169	3	0.018
19	167	7	0.042
20	169	5	0.030
21	171	4	0.023
22	170	3	0.018

observed rates and corresponding control limits are also depicted on the chart. During the first 10 months the process is in a state of statistical control since all observed fractions lie within the control limits. The fractions observed during the subsequent 12 months are also depicted on the control chart. It appears that following the intervention, the process gets out of control since all values lie below the centreline, and 6 of the 12 values lie below the lower control limit. During the last 12 months, 57 out of 2025 specimens were contaminated, giving an average contamination rate of 0.028.

Figure 2.11 (b) depicts the control chart calculated, using this $\hat{p}$ value and the corresponding 12 observed contamination rates. All values are within their control limits. These data support the contention that the intervention was successful since subsequent to the intervention the process has stabilised at a new and significantly lower level.

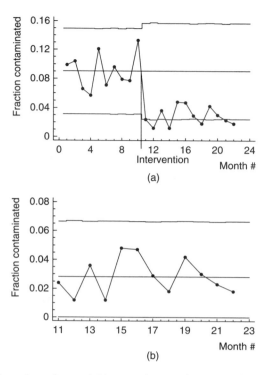

Figure 2.11 (a) p chart for variable sample size depicting the fraction of blood cultures that were contaminated as calculated for each of 22 months. The data of the first 10 months were used to calculate the chart. During the following 12 months the blood specimens for culture were obtained from a remote site. Previously it had been collected through a newly inserted intravenous catheter. (b) p chart for variable sample size depicting the fraction of blood cultures that were contaminated for each of 12 months following the introduction of a new procedure for collecting blood specimens for culture. The data depicted were used to calculate the chart. The process is in statistical control.

2.3.2 The u Chart

A u chart is used instead of the c chart to monitor the number of defects per inspection unit when the number of inspection units varies between samples. As for the c chart, we assume that the number of defects per inspection unit follows a Poisson distribution. The quantity u_i is the average number of defects per inspection unit in the ith sample. It is calculated as

$$u_i = \frac{\sum_{j=1}^{n_i} c_{ij}}{n_i} \qquad (2.39)$$

where c_{ij} is the number of defects of the jth inspection unit in the ith sample, and n_i is the number of inspection units in the ith sample. $\bar{u}$ is the weighted mean of u_i. It is calculated as

$$\bar{u} = \frac{\sum_{i=1}^{k} u_i n_i}{\sum_{i=1}^{k} n_i} = \frac{\sum_{i=1}^{k} \sum_{j=1}^{n_i} c_{ij}}{\sum_{i=1}^{k} n_i} \quad (2.40)$$

where k is the number of samples. The number of defects per inspection unit follows a Poisson distribution. Based on this assumption, it may be shown that the standard deviation of u_i can be estimated by

$$\hat{\sigma}_{u_i} = \sqrt{\frac{\bar{u}}{n_i}} \quad (2.41)$$

Therefore, the u chart has

$$\text{UCL}_i = \bar{u} + 3\sqrt{\frac{\bar{u}}{n_i}} \quad (2.42)$$

$$\text{centreline} = \bar{u} \quad (2.43)$$

$$\text{LCL}_i = \bar{u} - 3\sqrt{\frac{\bar{u}}{n_i}} \quad (2.44)$$

where UCL_i and LCL_i are the control limits of the ith sample.

The following example is constructed from data read from figures in a study by Greene *et al.* [10]. The data have been modified a little, but the main idea of the study has been maintained.

Example 2.10

Using a clinical information system, all episodes of acute sinusitis initiated between January 1, 1999 and October 31, 2000 within a community-wide individual practice association were identified. An episode of sinusitis was defined as the diagnosis, treatment, and care of a single patient, suffering from acute sinusitis. Each episode was evaluated in relation to a sinusitis care pathway based on the most important elements of evidence-based care such as use of proper first-line and second-line antibiotics, proper sequence of diagnostic and therapeutic procedures, etc. For each episode the information system generated the number of deviations from the care pathway. A deviation is referred to as an exception to recommended treatment and care in the following.

Table 2.10 shows for each month, the number of exceptions occurring, the number of episodes initiated, and exceptions per episode. A u chart may be constructed from the data. $\bar{u}$ is calculated as the total number of exceptions for the first 22 months (7216, see Table 2.10) divided by the total number of episodes (22 045, see Table 2.10) to obtain $\bar{u} = 0.327$ exception/month. Using this value and Equation (2.41), the standard deviation of each month may be calculated. For March 1999, e.g., the standard deviation is equal to $\sqrt{\frac{0.327}{1029}} = 0.018$. Therefore, the control limits for this month are $\bar{u} \pm 3\hat{\sigma}_{u_i} = 0.327 \pm 0.054 = 0.273$ to 0.381. The observed number of exceptions per episode for this month (0.343) is within the control limits.

Figure 2.12 (a) shows the u chart. The observed exceptions per episode are also depicted on the chart. It appears that the process is in statistical control up to and including month # 22, i.e., October 2000.

At this time, a multifaceted intervention program was initiated, consisting of physician education, a locally developed sinusitis care pathway (see above), feedback through a physician profiling system, financial incentives, and patient education. To assess the impact of this program, the exceptions per episode was calculated for each month covering the period January, 2001 to December 31, 2001. These results are also shown in Table 2.10. The number of exception per month, during this period, has been depicted in Figure 2.12 (a). It appears that following the initiation of the intervention program and contrary to the prior stable state during the previous 22 months, the process gets out of statistical control. Figure 2.12 (b) shows a u chart calculated from the data recorded during the last 12 months of the period, following the start of the intervention. Now the process has stabilised at a significantly lower level.

2.3.3 The $\overline{X}$ Chart and the S Chart

When the sample size varies, $\hat{\mu}$ and $\overline{S}$ as estimators of μ and σ are calculated using weighted sample values, as follows

$$\hat{\mu} = \frac{\sum\limits_{i=1}^{k} n_i \overline{X}_i}{\sum\limits_{i=1}^{k} n_i} \qquad (2.45)$$

Table 2.10 Number of exceptions from sinusitis pathway, number of sinusitis episodes initiated, and exceptions per episode on each of 34 consecutive months. Following month # 22 a multifaceted intervention program was initiated (intervention).

Month/year	Number of exceptions	Number of episodes	Exceptions per episode
1/99	363	1010	0.359
2/99	345	1005	0.343
3/99	353	1029	0.343
4/99	308	997	0.309
5/99	280	980	0.286
6/99	300	1001	0.300
7/99	315	1021	0.309
8/99	335	995	0.337
9/99	295	998	0.296
10/99	337	977	0.345
11/99	365	988	0.369
12/99	345	1021	0.338
1/00	360	994	0.362
2/00	337	989	0.341
3/00	322	1021	0.315
4/00	312	1011	0.309
5/00	350	973	0.360
6/00	360	1027	0.351
7/00	320	998	0.321
8/00	322	1019	0.316
9/00	285	992	0.287
10/00	312	999	0.312
Intervention			
11/00	325	998	0.326
12/00	300	994	0.302
1/01	263	995	0.264
2/01	245	997	0.246
3/01	285	1009	0.283
4/01	230	994	0.231
5/01	215	1022	0.210
6/01	234	1018	0.230
7/01	220	1015	0.217
8/01	237	981	0.242
9/01	220	997	0.221
10/01	230	1000	0.230
11/01	272	996	0.273
12/01	270	1022	0.264

First 22 months: 22 045 episodes and 7216 exceptions.
Last 12 months: 12 046 episodes and 2921 exceptions.

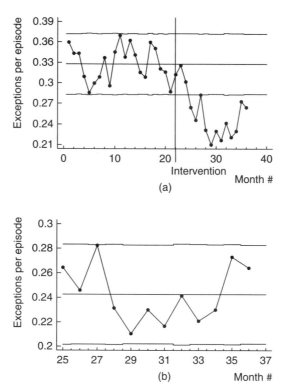

Figure 2.12 (a) u chart depicting the number of exceptions from a sinusitis care pathway per sinusitis episode initiated per month for each of 36 consecutive months. The u chart was calculated using the data of the first 22 months; at the end of this period a multifaceted intervention program was initiated. (b) u chart depicting the number of exceptions from a sinusitis care pathway per sinusitis episode initiated per month, for each of the last 12 of the 36 months depicted in Figure 2.12 (a). Two months prior to the start of the present series a multifaceted intervention program had been initiated (see Figure 2.12 (a)). The u chart was calculated using the data depicted on the chart. It appears that the process has stabilized at a new and improved level, relative to that of the first 22 months.

where $\overline{X}_i$ is the mean of the ith sample, n_i its size, and k the number of samples, and

$$\overline{S} = \sqrt{\frac{\sum_{i=1}^{k} S_i^2 (n_i - 1)}{\sum_{i=1}^{k} (n_i - 1)}} = \sqrt{\frac{\sum_{i=1}^{k} \sum_{j=1}^{n_i} (X_{ij} - \overline{X}_i)^2}{\sum_{i=1}^{k} n_i - k}} \qquad (2.46)$$

where S_i is the standard deviation of the ith sample.

The control limits of the $\overline{X}$ chart are defined by

$$\hat{\mu} \pm 3 \frac{\overline{S}}{c_4(h)\sqrt{n_i}} \tag{2.47}$$

where $h = \sum_{i=1}^{k} n_i - k + 1$ and $c_4(h) = c_4$ is defined in Section 1.2 and its approximate value can be found in Table 1.1 under $n = h$.

The S chart does not have a centreline because the expected value of the standard deviation depends on the sample size. Instead the expected value (the centre point) is calculated as follows

$$\text{Centre point} = c_4(n_i) \frac{\overline{S}}{c_4(h)} \tag{2.48}$$

when σ is unknown. The upper control limit of the ith sample is given by

$$\text{UCL} = \frac{c_4(n_i)\overline{S}}{c_4(h)} \left(1 + 3 \frac{\sqrt{1 - c_4^2(n_i)}}{c_4(n_i)} \right) \tag{2.49}$$

The corresponding lower limit is given by

$$\text{LCL} = \max\left\{ 0; \frac{c_4(n_i)\overline{S}}{c_4(h)} \left(1 - 3 \frac{\sqrt{1 - c_4^2(n_i)}}{c_4(n_i)} \right) \right\} \tag{2.50}$$

These equations are derived in appendix B.

Example 2.11

This example was inspired by the study by Nizard et al. [11]. We used the distribution of their data (see Table 1 in their paper). However, the time sequence we have used is different from theirs, and the splitting of the data into weekly samples is our own invention.

At an orthopaedic department a computer tomography-based navigation system for total knee replacement (TKR) was introduced. This
technique was applied in 78 consecutive patients who had TKR of one
or both knees due to osteoarthritis or rheumatoid arthritis. Several outcome measures were recorded. Here, we will focus on the alignment (the
angle of the femuro-tibial axis). The target value was 180°, and the
specification interval was 180° ± 3°.

Table 2.11 shows, for each of 19 consecutive weeks, the number of
TKRs performed, the mean and standard deviation of the corresponding
alignments, the expected standard deviation (the centre point), and the
UCL and LCL of the mean as well as of the standard deviation. Using
Equations (2.45) and (2.46), the grand mean and the pooled standard
deviation were calculated as

$$\hat{\mu} = \frac{3 \cdot 178.33 + 5 \cdot 178.60 + \ldots + 4 \cdot 180.75}{3 + 5 + \ldots + 4} = 180.15$$

Table 2.11 Sample size, mean, standard deviation, upper (UCL), and lower (LCL)
control limits for the $\overline{X}$ chart and S chart, and centre point for the S chart of each of
19 samples of alignment measurements made in patients following total knee replacement operation.

Sample #	n	Sample mean	Sample standard deviation	LCL for $\overline{X}$ chart	UCL for $\overline{X}$ chart	Centre point for S chart	LCL for S chart	UCL for S chart
1	3	178.33	3.21	176.19	184.11	2.02	0	5.20
2	5	178.60	3.13	177.09	183.22	2.15	0	4.49
3	2	179.00	2.83	175.29	185.01	1.82	0	5.96
4	4	177.25	2.63	176.72	183.58	2.11	0	4.77
5	3	179.00	2.00	176.19	184.11	2.03	0	5.20
6	6	180.33	2.66	177.35	182.95	2.18	0.07	4.28
7	5	181.60	0.89	177.09	183.22	2.15	0	4.49
8	5	179.40	1.52	177.09	183.22	2.15	0	4.49
9	4	180.00	1.83	176.72	183.58	2.11	0	4.77
10	8	180.88	2.17	177.73	182.58	2.21	0.41	4.00
11	5	181.40	1.52	177.09	183.22	2.15	0	4.49
12	3	181.33	2.89	176.19	184.11	2.03	0	5.20
13	4	180.00	2.16	176.72	183.58	2.10	0	4.77
14	4	180.75	2.87	176.72	183.58	2.10	0	4.77
15	3	178.33	0.58	176.19	184.11	2.03	0	5.20
16	5	181.40	2.19	177.09	183.22	2.15	0	4.49
17	3	181.33	2.08	176.19	184.11	2.03	0	5.20
18	2	181.50	2.12	175.30	185.00	1.82	0	5.96
19	4	180.75	2.63	176.72	183.58	2.11	0	4.77

and

$$\overline{S} = \sqrt{\frac{3.21^2 \cdot 2 + 3.13^2 \cdot 4 + \ldots + 2.63^2 \cdot 3}{(3 + 5 + \ldots + 4) - 19}} = 2.28,$$

respectively, $h = \sum_{j=1}^{k} n_j - k + 1 = 60$. From the approximation formula in Table 1.1,

$$c_4(h) = c_4(60) = 0.9958.$$

Using Equation (2.47), UCL and LCL of the $\overline{X}$ chart may be calculated for each of the 19 samples. For sample # 4, e.g., the control limits of the $\overline{X}$ chart are calculated as

$$180.15 \pm \frac{3 \cdot 2.28}{0.9958\sqrt{4}} = 180.15 \pm 3.43$$

giving UCL $= 183.58$ and LCL $= 176.72$. The centre point of sample # 4 for the S chart is calculated using Table 1.1 and Equation (2.50) as

$$c_4(n_i)\frac{\overline{S}}{c_4(h)} = \frac{2.28 \cdot 0.9213}{0.9958} = 2.111$$

where $c_4(4) = 0.9213$ and $c_4(60) = 0.9958$. Using Equation (2.49) the UCL is calculated as

$$\frac{c(n_i)\overline{S}}{c_4(h)}\left(1 + 3\frac{\sqrt{1 - c_4^2(n_i)}}{c_4(n_i)}\right) = \frac{0.9213 \cdot 2.28}{0.9958}\left(1 + 3\frac{\sqrt{1 - 0.9213^2}}{0.9213}\right) = 4.77$$

Using Equation (2.50) we find LCL $= 0$.

Figure 2.13 (a) shows the $\overline{X}$ chart and Figure 2.13 (b) shows the corresponding S chart. Judging from these results, we may conclude that the standard deviation, as well as the mean, is stable.

The reader may find additional examples of the practical application of control charts in the book by RG Carey and RC Lloyd [12] and the book by MK Hart and RF Hart [13].

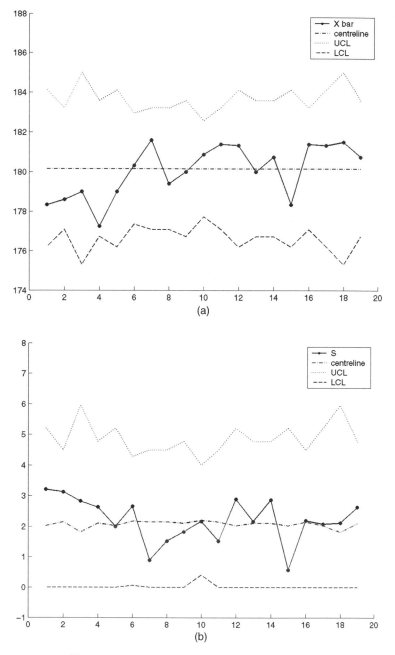

Figure 2.13 (a) $\overline{X}$ chart for unequal sample size depicting femuro-tibial axis/degree
(•-•-•). Legends for centreline, upper (UCL) and lower (LCL) control limit are shown
in Figure 2.13(b). (b) S chart for unequal sample size depicting observed sample
standard deviation (•-•-•) of femuro-tibial axis/degree.

REFERENCES

[1] Duncan AJ. Quality Control and Industrial Statistics. McGraw-hill, USA, 1986.

[2] Curran ET, Benneyan JC, and Hood J. Controlling methicillin-resistant staphylococcus aureus: a feedback approach using annotated statistical process control charts. Infect Control Hosp Epidemiol 2002; 23:13–8.

[3] Nelson FE, Hart MK, and Hart RF. Application of control chart statistics to blood pressure measurement variability in the primary care setting. J Am Acad Nurse Pract 1994; 6:17–28.

[4] Finison LJ, Finison KS, and Bliersbach CM. The use of control charts to improve healthcare quality. J Health Qual 1993; 15:9–23.

[5] Quesenberry CP. Statistical process control geometric Q-chart for nosocomial infection surveillance. Am J Infect Control 2000; 28:314–20.

[6] Montgomery DC. Introduction to Statistical Quality Control. Wiley and Sons Inc, New York, 2001.

[7] Boggs PB, Wheeler D, Washburne WF, and Hayati F. Peak expiratory flow rate control chart in asthma care: chart construction and use in asthma care. Ann Allergy Asthma Immunol 1998; 81:552–62.

[8] Fasting S, and Gisvold SE. Statistical process control methods allow the analysis and improvement of anesthesia care. Can J Anesth 2003; 50:767–74.

[9] Norberg A, Christopher NC, Ramundo ML, Bower JR, and Bermen SA. Contamination rates of blood cultures obtained by dedicated phlebotomy vs intravenous catheter. JAMA 2003; 289:726–9.

[10] Greene RA, Bechman H, Chamberlain J, Partridge G, Miller M, Burden D, and Kerr J. Increasing adherence to a community-based guideline for acute sinusitis through education, physician profiling, and financial incentives. Am J Manag Care 2004; 10:670–8.

[11] Nizard RS, Porcher R, Ravaud P, Vangaver E, Hannouche D, Bizot P, and Sedel L. Use of the cusum technique for evaluation of a CT-based navigation system for total knee replacement. Clin Orthop Relat R 2004; 425:180–8.

[12] Carey RG, and Lloyd RC. Measuring Quality Improvement in Healthcare. A Guide to Statistical Process Control Applications. Quality Press, Milwaukee, Wisconsin, 2001.

[13] Hart MK, and Hart RF. Statistical Process Control for Health Care. Duxbury, California, 2002.

3

Time-Weighted Control Charts

3.1 SHORTCOMINGS OF SHEWHART CHARTS

In Chapters 1 and 2, Shewhart charts were introduced. Shewhart charts, especially the $\overline{X}$ chart and the X chart, have been used widely for monitoring the process mean in industry. However, these charts have shortcomings. In Chapter 1, the average run length (ARL) was introduced as a performance criterion for control charts. The run length is the number of observations that must be plotted before an observation indicates an out-of-control condition. For an ideal chart, when the mean of a process has not changed, the ARL should be large, and when the mean changes, the ARL should be small to quickly indicate this change. When the process variable follows a Gaussian distribution, the in-control ARL for an X chart with 3σ limits is 370, and when the mean has changed by 0.5 standard deviation, the out-of-control ARL is 155. So when the process is in statistical control, the X chart will signal a false alarm after 370 observations, on average, and when the process mean has changed by 0.5 σ, the X chart will not give a warning until after 155 observations, on average. Column 2 of Table 3.1 lists the ARL for an X chart corresponding to various step changes of the mean, shown in the first column.

Each ARL was calculated based on the corresponding probability distribution. Obviously, the X chart can quickly detect large (2 and 3σ) step changes of the mean, but it is not sensitive to small step changes. Simulations were used to obtain the ARLs for the other two control charts, by repeatedly generating independent observations, all following the same Gaussian distribution. For details see the legend for Table 3.1.

Statistical Development of Quality in Medicine   P. Winkel and N. F. Zhang
© 2007 John Wiley & Sons, Ltd

Table 3.1 Average run length (ARL) for X, cumulative sum (CUSUM), and exponentially weighted moving average (EWMA) charts in the presence of various changes in the mean value of the process. For the X chart, the ARL was calculated, and for the two other charts, it was determined using simulation experiments.

In each experiment, a time series of data was generated by simulation using a Gaussian distribution with standard deviation of 1.0 and initial mean of 0.0, and a control chart was constructed, using these data. Then the mean of the Gaussian distribution was changed and the run length recorded. This experiment was repeated at least 2000 times for each change of the mean and each type of control chart, and the ARL was computed. The parameters of the CUSUM and EWMA charts have been adjusted to give in-control ARL values approximately equal to that of the X chart.

Change of mean (the unit is 1 standard deviation)	X chart (parameter, $k = 3$)	CUSUM chart (parameters, $h = 4.76$, $k = 0.5$)	EWMA chart (parameters, $\lambda = 0.2$, $L = 2.87$)
0.0	370.37	374.66	370.01
0.5	155.21	35.48	36.05
1.0	43.89	9.91	9.59
2.0	6.30	3.84	3.53
3.0	2.00	2.49	2.27

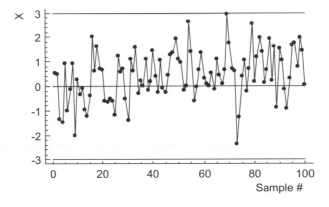

Figure 3.1 One hundred values were generated from Gaussian distributions and then depicted on a control chart with centreline = 0.00, upper control limit = 3.00, and lower control limit = −3.00 The mean of the distribution generating the first 30 values was 0.00, while the mean of that generating the remaining values was 0.50. In both cases the standard deviation was 1.00.

Example 3.1

Figure 3.1 shows an X chart with 3σ limits. The centreline is 0.0, and the standard deviation is 1.0. One hundred values are depicted on the chart. The values were generated by simulation using Gaussian distributions. The distribution generating the first 30 values had a mean value of 0.0, while that generating the remaining values had a mean value of 0.5. In both cases the standard deviation was 1.0. Visually, we note a change in the location of the values following the increase in the mean of the distribution generating the values. However, the last 70 values are all within the control limits of the control chart. Therefore, the X chart cannot detect a small mean shift such as 0.5σ in this data set.

3.2   CUMULATIVE SUM CHARTS

To improve the detection capability relative to that of the Shewhart control charts, several control charts have been developed. Among them, the cumulative sum (CUSUM) and the exponentially weighted moving average (EWMA) charts are popular. Given a sequence of values $\{X_i\}$ generated from a process, a CUSUM statistic is formed by plotting the quantity

$$C_i = \sum_{j=1}^{i} (X_j - \mu_0) \qquad (3.1)$$

or the quantity

$$C_i = \sum_{j=1}^{i} \frac{X_j - \mu_0}{\sigma} \qquad (3.2)$$

where μ_0 is the process mean or a target value, σ is the process standard deviation. We assume that σ is known. Equation (3.2) is often referred to as the standardised CUSUM or scaled CUSUM. We will use Equation (3.1) for CUSUM charts. As long as the process remains in statistical control, the mean of C_i is 0. It may be shown that the variance of C_i in Equation (3.1) is $i\sigma^2$. The CUSUM statistic will show variation in a random pattern centred at 0 (but with increasing variations). If the process mean increases, the charted CUSUM points will eventually drift upwards, and vice versa, if it decreases. Therefore, if a significant trend develops, we should consider this as evidence that the process mean has changed, and a search for some assignable cause should be performed.

CUSUM charts were first proposed by Page (1954) [1] and have been studied by many authors. Early medical applications include [2–4]. The tabular form of the CUSUM is based on Wald's sequential test (see Chapter 6 on risk adjusted control charts), that is used to choose between two competing hypotheses. For a specified type of outcome measure, a quantity (W_j) is repeatedly calculated and used to update a cumulated sum S_j. This quantity depends on two competing hypotheses and the observed outcome. The initial value of the sum (S_0) is usually set equal to 0.

We have

$$S_i = \sum_{j=1}^{i} W_j \qquad (3.3)$$

where W_j is the value corresponding to the jth observation. It has been shown that the optimal choice for W_j to discriminate between the two hypotheses is based on the log-likelihood ratio [5, 6]. We have

$$W_j = \log\left(\frac{L_{1,j}}{L_{0,j}}\right) \qquad (3.4)$$

where $L_{0,j}$ and $L_{1,j}$ are the likelihood functions based on the hypotheses H_0 and H_1. For example, assume the null hypothesis is $H_0 : \mu = \mu_0$ and the alternative hypothesis is $H_1 : \mu = \mu_1$. This corresponds to testing if the process mean has changed from μ_0 to μ_1. When the process variable X_j follows a Gaussian distribution, the log-likelihood ratio W_j in Equation (3.4) is equal to $2X_j(\mu_1 - \mu_0) + (\mu_0^2 - \mu_1^2)$, which is equivalent to

$$X_j - \mu_0 - \frac{\mu_1 - \mu_0}{2} \qquad (3.5)$$

$K = \frac{\mu_1 - \mu_0}{2}$ is called a reference value.

The CUSUM chart may be designed to detect a positive deviation or a negative deviation from the process mean μ_0. It is assumed that the standard deviation of the process does not change. Assume that we want to detect a step change of the process mean to a value of μ_1 ($\mu_1 > \mu_0$). To do so, we cumulate the deviation of each observation (X_j) from the mean μ_0, i.e., ($X_j - \mu_0$). The Expression (3.5) becomes positive if X_j is closer to μ_1 than to μ_0. This follows because $\frac{\mu_1 - \mu_0}{2}$ is the median between the two values. Therefore, positive deviations are in favour of the hypothesis that the mean = μ_1. By contrast, negative deviations are in favour of the hypothesis that the mean = μ_0. The slack value, k, is the median value in the unit of one standard deviation, i.e., $k = \frac{K}{\sigma} = \frac{\mu_1 - \mu_0}{2\sigma}$. Thus, Expression (3.5) can be written as $X_i - \mu_0 - k\sigma$. We define a function of the sample number, i, as

$$S_+(i) = \max\{0; S_+(i-1) + X_i - \mu_0 - k\sigma\} \qquad (3.6)$$

This quantity is depicted on a CUSUM chart designed to detect an increase in the process mean value. The following quantity is depicted on a CUSUM chart designed to detect a decrease in the process mean (a change to a value that is $< \mu_0$)

$$S_-(i) = \max\{0; S_-(i-1) - X_i + \mu_0 - k\sigma\} \qquad (3.7)$$

The two charts may be combined into a single chart by plotting $S_+(i)$ above the line $Y = 0$ and $-S_-(i)$ below this line.

The initial values of these two functions are usually set to 0, i.e., $S_+(0) = S_-(0) = 0$. Having defined the function that we want to monitor, we need to define a control limit (H). This is defined as a multiple (h) of the process standard deviation (σ). We have

$$H = h \cdot \sigma \qquad (3.8)$$

The parameter H is often called the decision interval. If either $S_+(i)$ or $S_-(i)$ is larger than H the process is assumed to be out of control. The choice of the parameters h and k determines the performance of the CUSUM chart. It has been recommended [7] that using $h = 4$ to 5 and $k = 0.5$ (which corresponds to $\mu_1 - \mu_0 = \sigma$) will generally provide a CUSUM chart that has good ARL properties, against a shift of about 1σ in the process mean. In Table 3.1, the ARLs of the CUSUM chart with $h = 4.76$ and $k = 0.5$ are listed for step changes of the process mean of 0.0, 0.5, 1.0, 2.0, and 3.0 in the unit of process standard deviation, σ. Based on simulation, it is found that the in-control ARL of the CUSUM chart is 374.66, which is comparable to 370.37, the in-control ARL of the X chart. By contrast, the out-of-control ARLs of the CUSUM chart are smaller than those of the X chart for changes in the process mean of 0.5, 1.0, and 2.0σ.

For illustration, we applied the tabular CUSUM chart to the data shown in Figure 3.1. With $h = 5$ and $k = 0.5$, a CUSUM chart is designed to detect a change in the process mean of 1σ.

Figure 3.2 shows a CUSUM chart based on a process mean of 0.0 and a process standard deviation of 1.0 with upper control limit = 5.0 and

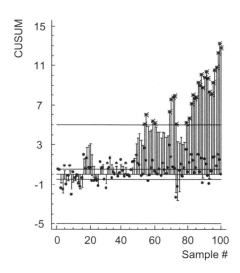

Figure 3.2 One hundred values, generated from a Gaussian distribution, were used as input to a CUSUM chart, designed to detect a mean shift of 1.00 standard deviation, while the in-control mean of the process variable is 0.00 and its standard deviation is 1.00. $h = 5.00$ and $k = 0.50$. $S_+(i)$ and $-S_-(i)$ are depicted on the chart (the bars). The deviation of each observation from the target value 0.00 is also shown (the dots). The mean of the distribution generating the first 30 values was 0.00, while the mean of that generating the remaining values was 0.50. In both cases the standard deviation was 1.00.

lower control limit $= -5.0$. $S_+(i)$ and $-S_-(i)$ are depicted on the chart. Thirty values are outside the control limits, starting from observation number 54. The process mean was increased after sample number 30. Therefore, the run length is $54 - 30 = 24$, as opposed to at least 70 with the X chart (see Figure 3.1).

The major advantage of using CUSUM charts relative to the Shewhart charts is that the former are more effective in detecting small shifts in the process mean as indicated in Table 3.1 and illustrated in the above example. The CUSUM chart also has another advantage. From the Central Limit Theorem it follows that the cumulative sum with a large number of observations will follow an approximate Gaussian distribution even if the distribution of the process variable deviates considerably from a Gaussian one. A disadvantage of the CUSUM chart is that it is not as effective as the X chart in detecting large transient changes in the process mean. Therefore, it is recommended to use a CUSUM chart together with a Shewhart chart. One may add that the CUSUM chart is not a very effective procedure for analysing and diagnosing past data because the cumulative sums are correlated.

Thus, contrary to the case for the X chart, systematic patterns of data, e.g., long sequences above the centreline, cannot be used to diagnose why a process is out of control.

To construct a standardised CUSUM chart (see Equation (3.2)), we first define

$$Y_i = \frac{X_i - \mu}{\sigma}$$

The standardised CUSUM charts are constructed by plotting

$$S'_+(i) = \max\{0; S'_+(i-1) + Y_i - k\} \tag{3.9}$$

and

$$S'_-(i) = \max\{0; S'_-(i-1) - Y_i - k\} \tag{3.10}$$

The recommended values of the parameters h and k are the same as for the nonstandardised charts.

Example 3.2

In Example 2.11 we examined the alignment (the angle of the femuro-tibial axis) as a measure of the outcome of a total knee replacement (TKR) using a computer tomography-based navigation system in 78 consecutive patients. The target value was 180°. The mean of the 78 values was 180.18°, and the standard deviation was 2.038°. Assume we want to detect a change of 1 standard deviation, $\mu_1 - \mu_0 = 1\sigma$. The slack value k will be 0.5. The target value is set equal to 180°.

Table 3.2 shows X_i, $X_i - 180 - 0.5\sigma$, $S_-(i)$, $180 - X_i - 0.5\sigma$, and $S_+(i)$ for the first 20 observations. For example, for X_1 we obtain the following values, $(X_1 - 180) - 0.5\sigma = (176 - 180) - 1.019 = -5.019°$, $S_-(1) = \max\{0; -5.019 + S_-(0)\} = \max\{0; -5.019 + 0.000\} = 0°$, $(180 - X_1) - 0.5\sigma = (180 - 176) - 1.019 = 2.981°$, and $S_+(1) = \max\{0; 2.981 + S_+(0)\} = \max\{0; 2.981 + 0.000\} = 2.981°$, etc. For the upper and lower control limits, we choose $h = 5.0$. They are $5.0 \cdot 2.038° = 10.19°$ and $-5 \cdot 2.038° = -10.19°$ respectively. Figure 3.3 shows $S_+(i)$ and $-S_-(i)$ of all 78 values.

For comparison $X_i - 180°$, the observed deviations from the target, are also shown.

Table 3.2 $S_-(i)$ and $S_+(i)$ calculated for the first 20 values of $X_i =$ (angle of the femuro-tibial axis)/degree as measured in patients following total knee replacement. The target value is 180, and the standard deviation is 2.038.

i	X_i	$180 - X_i - k\sigma$	$S_-(i) =$ max $\{0; S_-(i-1)+$ $180 - X_i - k\sigma\}$	$X_i - 180 - k\sigma$	$S_+(i) =$ max $\{0; S_+(i-1)+$ $X_i - 180 - k\sigma\}$
1	176	+2.981	+2.981	−5.019	0.000
2	177	+1.981	+4.962	−4.019	0.000
3	182	−3.019	+1.943	+0.981	+0.981
4	182	+3.019	0.000	+0.981	+1.962
5	176	+2.981	+2.981	−5.019	0.000
6	177	+1.981	+4.962	−4.019	0.000
7	182	−3.019	+1.943	+0.981	+0.981
8	176	+2.981	+4.924	−5.019	0.000
9	181	−2.019	+2.905	−0.019	0.000
10	177	+1.981	+4.886	−4.019	0.000
11	177	+1.981	+6.867	−4.019	0.000
12	181	−2.019	+4.849	−0.019	0.000
13	175	+3.981	+8.829	−6.019	0.000
14	176	+2.981	+11.810	−5.019	0.000
15	179	−0.019	+11.791	−2.019	0.000
16	177	+1.981	+13.772	−4.019	0.000
17	181	−2.019	+11.753	−0.019	0.000
18	177	+1.981	+13.734	−4.019	0.000
19	177	+1.981	+15.715	−4.019	0.000
20	183	−4.019	+11.696	+1.981	+1.981

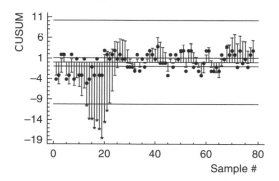

Figure 3.3 Seventy-eight values of (angle of the femuro-tibial axis)/degree, measured in patients following total knee replacement, were input to a CUSUM chart. The target value of the chart is 180.00, and the standard deviation is 2.04. The chart is designed to detect a change in the mean of ±1.00 standard deviation with $h = 5.00$ and $k = 0.50$. $S_+(i)$ and $-S_-(i)$ are depicted on the chart (the bars or stars when outside the control limits). The deviation of each observation from the target value 180.00 is also shown (the dots).

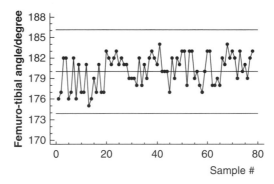

Figure 3.4 Seventy-eight values of (angle of the femuro-tibial axis)/degree, measured in patients following total knee replacement, are depicted on an X chart. The values were used to calculate the X chart. k, the parameter of the X chart, is 3.00.

Figure 3.4 shows the corresponding X chart where the target is 180° and the process standard deviation is 2.038°. Contrary to the X chart, the CUSUM chart for individual values showed that initially the process was not in control, probably due to a learning effect. If one discards the first 20 observations and depicts the remaining ones on a CUSUM chart (not shown), the standard deviation drops to 1.758°, and all CUSUM values are well within the control limits.

3.3   EXPONENTIALLY WEIGHTED MOVING AVERAGE (EWMA) CHARTS

The EWMA chart was introduced by Roberts (1959) [8]. See also Hunter (1986) [9] for a good discussion of the EWMA. For a sequence of observations of X_i with mean μ and variance σ^2, the EWMA statistic is defined as

$$Z_i = (1 - \lambda)Z_{i-1} + \lambda X_i \tag{3.11}$$

where $i = 1, 2, \ldots$, λ is a parameter ($0 < \lambda \leq 1$), and the starting value $Z_0 = \mu$, the process mean. It may be shown that

$$Z_i = \lambda \sum_{j=0}^{i-1} [(1 - \lambda)^j X_{i-j}] + (1 - \lambda)^i \mu \tag{3.12}$$

Therefore, Z_i is a weighted average of the X_j ($j = 1, \ldots, i$) and μ with the weights of X_j decreasing exponentially. The weight of the current observation is λ, that of the previous one is $\lambda(1 - \lambda)$, etc. The older the observation is, the smaller the value will be $\lambda(1 - \lambda)^j$ with which it is weighted. It may be shown that the variance of Z_i is

$$\left(\frac{\lambda}{2 - \lambda}\right)[1 - (1 - \lambda)^{2i}]\sigma^2 \tag{3.13}$$

When i is large, an approximate variance is

$$\left(\frac{\lambda}{2 - \lambda}\right)\sigma^2 \tag{3.14}$$

An EWMA chart can be established by plotting Z_i with the centreline at μ or a target value. The control limits are based on Equation (3.13). We have

$$\text{UCL}_i = \mu + L\sigma\sqrt{\frac{\lambda}{2 - \lambda}[1 - (1 - \lambda)^{2i}]} \tag{3.15}$$

$$\text{centreline} = \mu \tag{3.16}$$

$$\text{LCL}_i = \mu - L\sigma\sqrt{\frac{\lambda}{2 - \lambda}[1 - (1 - \lambda)^{2i}]} \tag{3.17}$$

where L is a parameter. When $i > 10$, Equation (3.14) may be used to obtain the control limits

$$\text{UCL} = \mu + L\sigma\sqrt{\frac{\lambda}{2 - \lambda}} \tag{3.18}$$

and

$$\text{LCL} = \mu - L\sigma\sqrt{\frac{\lambda}{2 - \lambda}} \tag{3.19}$$

For illustration, the EWMA chart is applied to the data depicted in Figure 3.1 with $\lambda = 0.2$ and $L = 3$ assuming a process mean of 0.0 and standard deviation of 1.0. The UCL and LCL are based on the approximation formulae in (3.18) and (3.19).

The result is shown in Figure 3.5. Eight points are outside the control limits, starting from the observation number 55. The mean of the distribution, generating the data depicted on the chart, changed from 0.0 to 0.5 after the first 30 values had been generated while its standard

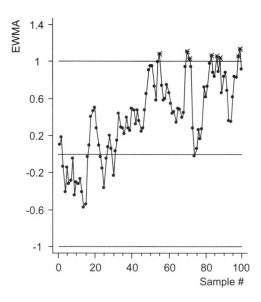

Figure 3.5   One hundred values, generated from Gaussian distributions, were used as input to an EWMA chart with target value = 0.00, λ = 0.20, and L = 3.00. The mean of the distribution generating the first 30 values was 0.0, while the mean of that generating the remaining values was 0.50. In both cases the standard deviation was 1.00.

deviation remained equal to 1.0. Therefore, the run length of the EWMA is $55 - 30 = 25$.

When the X chart is used, the out-of-control condition (a value outside the control limits) depends only on the current value. By contrast, when the EWMA chart is used, the out-of-control condition depends on Z_i, which is an exponentially weighted average of the current and all prior values. After a while the weight of a given observation assumes a value that for all practical purposes is 0 (see Equation (3.12)). Therefore, it is outdated in the sense that it no longer impacts on the value of Z_i. The time elapsed before this to happen depends on the value of λ. $\lambda = 1$ implies that only the current measurement influences the EWMA. Therefore, in this case the EWMA chart becomes an X chart. One may increase the sensitivity of the EWMA chart by decreasing the value of λ, and vice versa.

The properties of the distribution of the run lengths of the EWMA chart have been studied. These studies provide tables of ARL for a range of values of λ and L. To design an EWMA chart one specifies the in-control ARL, the out-of-control ARL, and the magnitude of the change of the process mean important to detect. Then one selects the combination of λ and L that provide (approximately) the desired ARL performance given the change deemed important to detect. In general, it has been found that values of λ in the interval of $0.05 \leq \lambda \leq 0.25$ work well in practice, with $\lambda = 0.1$ and 0.2 being popular choices. It has also been found that $L = 3$ (the usual 3 sigma limits) works well.

Table 3.1 shows the value of the ARL of an EWMA chart with $\lambda = 0.2$ and $L = 2.87$ as a function of various step changes of the mean value of the process. For comparison, corresponding ARL values are shown for the X chart and the CUSUM chart. Like the CUSUM chart, the EWMA chart performs well against small to medium sized step changes of the process mean value. However, it does not react to large changes quite as quickly as the X chart. The EWMA chart is often slightly superior to the CUSUM chart in the presence of large shifts in the mean value when $\lambda > 0.01$ (see [7, p 432]). In addition, the EWMA chart has the advantage that the current EWMA value provides a forecast of the process mean value at the subsequent sample time [10, p 124]. The combined use of an X chart and an EWMA chart improves the sensitivity of the control procedure to large transient changes of the process mean without sacrificing its ability to detect smaller shifts quickly. It is possible to plot both X_i and Z_i on the same control chart [11].

Example 3.3

In Example 2.6, we examined the time between consecutive *Clostridium difficile* infections as a measure of the rate of infection. The distribution was definitely not Gaussian and we, therefore, transformed the values, using Nelson's transformation $Y = X^{0.2777}$ [12], but other approaches are also possible [13]. The distribution of the transformed data did not deviate significantly from a Gaussian distribution. Therefore, we depicted the values on an X chart, using the first six values to calculate the chart (see Figure 2.8).

Figure 3.6 shows the data depicted on a combined X-EWMA chart. The UCL and LCL are based on (3.18) and (3.19). It is noted that the EWMA detects a small decrease in the mean value that was not picked up by the X chart. Conversely, the large increase in the mean value was picked up by the X chart, but missed by the EWMA chart. This illustrates how the two charts complement each other. Large, but transient changes in the mean value are missed by the EWMA chart, but picked up by the X chart. Small but persistent changes in the mean value are picked up by the EWMA chart, but may go unnoticed for a long period if the X chart is used alone.

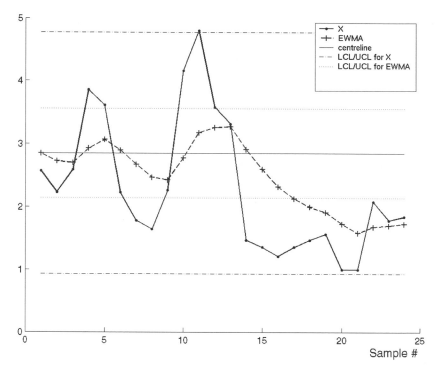

Figure 3.6 The time/day (X) between consecutive *Clostridium difficile* infections transformed using the transformation $Y = X^{0.2777}$ and then depicted on an X chart. The initial six transformed values were used to calculate the X chart k, the parameter of the X chart is 3.00. Superimposed on this chart is the corresponding exponentially weighted moving average (EWMA) chart with $\lambda = 0.20$ and $L = 3.00$. UCL is upper control limit and LCL is lower control limit.

REFERENCES

[1] Page ES. Continuous inspection schemes. Biometrika 1954; 41: 100–15.
[2] DeLeval MR, Francois K, Bull C, Brawn W and Spiegelhalter D. Analysis of a cluster of surgical failures. Application to a series of neonatal arterial switch operations. J Thorac Cardiovasc Surg 1994; 107:914–23.
[3] Williams SM, Parry BR and Schlup MTM. Quality control: an application of the cusum. BMJ 1992; 304:1359–61.
[4] Kinsey SE, Giles FJ and Holton J. Cusum plotting of temperature charts for assessing antimicrobial treatment in neutropenic patients. BMJ 1989; 299:775–6.
[5] Moustakides GV. Optimal stopping times for detecting changes in distributions. Ann Stat 1986; 14:1379–87.
[6] Steiner SH, Cook RJ, Farewell VT and Treasure T. Monitoring surgical performance using risk-adjusted cumulative sum charts. Biostatistics 2000; 1:441–52.

[7] Montgomery DC. Introduction to Statistical Quality Control, Wiley and Sons Inc, New York, 2001.

[8] Roberts SW. Control chart tests based on geometric moving averages. Technometrics 1959; 1: 239–51.

[9] Hunter JS. The exponentially weighted moving averages. J Qual Technol 1986; 18:203–10.

[10] Ryan TP. Statistical Methods for Quality Improvement. Wiley and Sons Inc, New York, 1989.

[11] Morton AP, Whitby M, McLaws M, Dobson A, McElwain S, Looke D and Stack-elroth J. The application of statistical process control charts to the detection and monitoring of hospital-acquired infections. J Qual Clin Practice 2001; 21:112–7.

[12] Nelson LS. A control chart for parts-per-million nonconforming items. J Qual Technol 1994; 26:239–40.

[13] Spliid H. Monitoring medical procedures by exponential smoothing. Stat Med 2006; (in press).

4

Control Charts for Autocorrelated Data

In Chapters 1, 2, and 3, Shewhart charts and other control charts were introduced for monitoring process mean and process variance. A basic assumption for applying these statistical process control charts is the independence of the process measurements. In this chapter, we focus on continuous process variables, define more precisely what independency actually means, and present various tests of the assumption of independency. To do so, we need to introduce the concept of a time series of observations generated by the process that we want to study. A time series may be viewed as the values taken on by a series of random variables observed at different times. We will refer to a random variable belonging to such a series as X_t where the index indicates the sequence number of the variable. The first variable in the sequence is X_1, the second one X_2 etc. The sequences of measurements dealt with so far in this book were assumed to have been generated by a sequence of random variables that all follow the same distribution and are independent of each other. Thus introducing the more complex concept of a time series was not necessary until now.

A series of random variables may be categorised as stationary or nonstationary [1, p 23–6]. The latter type is characterised among other things by the random variables not all having the same mean and/or variance. Furthermore, the dependencies among the variables may not be simple. This is an indication that the underlying process is not in statistical control. The topic here, however, is to identify dependency between observations generated by processes that are in statistical control. Therefore, the focus is on stationary

Statistical Development of Quality in Medicine   P. Winkel and N. F. Zhang
© 2007 John Wiley & Sons, Ltd

time series. In section 4.1 we will introduce the concept of a stationary time series. In section 4.2 we will introduce various tests that may be used to assess if the variables of a stationary sequence are independent of each other.

Dependency among observations impacts on the performance of the classical control charts for continuous data. In Section 4.3 we deal with this topic and introduce alternative control charts. In Section 4.4 we show how the choice of process standard deviation estimator impacts on the performance of the control charts in the presence of autocorrelation.

4.1 TIME SERIES ANALYSIS

A series of measurements obtained from a process during some period is a time series. In the following, we will assume that the period between consecutive measurements is approximately constant. The length of this period we shall refer to as a time unit. A time series $x_1, x_2, \ldots, x_n, \ldots$ can be viewed as the values taken on by a sequence of random variables $X_1, X_2, \ldots, X_n, \ldots$ or $\{X_t, t = 1, \ldots, n, \ldots\}$. The sequence $x_1, x_2, \ldots, x_n, \ldots$ is called a realization of $X_1, X_2, \ldots, X_n, \ldots$. We use the term time series to mean both the sequence of random variables $X_1, X_2, \ldots, X_n, \ldots$ and its realization. The sequence is stationary if it is in a state of 'statistical equilibrium'. This implies that the basic behaviour of the time series does not change in time. In particular, the time series $\{X_t\}$ have identical means and identical variances. The process corresponding to a stationary sequence of random variables is referred to as a stationary process.

4.1.1 Autocovariance and Autocorrelation

To examine the dependency between two random variables in a stationary sequence of random variables, we introduce the concept of covariance between two random variables that are a specified number of time units (τ) away from each other. It is defined as follows

$$\gamma(\tau) = \text{Cov}(X_i, X_j) = E[(X_i - \mu)(X_j - \mu)] \qquad (4.1)$$

where $j = i + \tau$ and μ is the mean of the stationary process. When X_i and X_j ($i \neq j$) are independent from each other, the covariance between them is zero. Therefore, when the covariance is not zero, the two random variables are dependent. Strictly speaking, two random variables with zero covariance are not necessarily independent. However, when both of them follow Gaussian distributions the statement is true.

Equivalent to the covariance, the correlation coefficient between two random variables is often used to measure their linear dependency. The correlation coefficient is defined as

$$\rho(\tau) = \rho_{ij} = \frac{\text{Cov}(X_i, X_j)}{\sigma_i \sigma_j} \tag{4.2}$$

where $j = i + \tau$, σ_i and σ_j are the standard deviations of X_i and X_j, respectively.

In a stationary sequence of random variables all pairs in the sequence that are separated by the same number of time units have identical covariances. Equations (4.1) and (4.2) apply to all pairs of variables separated by τ time units, i.e., for any i and $\tau = 0, \pm 1, \pm 2, \ldots$ For a stationary process, the covariance (correlation) between random variables one time unit apart is called the autocovariance (autocorrelation) of lag 1. In general the autocovariance (autocorrelation) between variables τ time units apart is called the autocovariance (autocorrelation) of lag τ.

For a stationary time series, $X_1, X_2, \ldots, X_n, \ldots$ if there exist nonzero $\rho(\tau)$ for any $\tau \neq 0$, then the sequence is called autocorrelated. For a stationary process, the autocorrelation of lag τ is

$$\rho(\tau) = \frac{\gamma(\tau)}{\sigma^2} \tag{4.3}$$

where σ^2 is the process variance. For a sequence, $X_1, X_2, \ldots, X_n$, the autocovariance at lag τ can be estimated by

$$\hat{\gamma}(\tau) = \frac{\sum_{i=1}^{n-\tau} (X_i - \overline{X})(X_{i+\tau} - \overline{X})}{n - \tau} \tag{4.4}$$

for $\tau = 0, 1, \ldots, n - 1$. In particular, when $\tau = 0$, $\hat{\gamma}(0)$ is an estimator of the process variance. In practice, the traditional sample variance S^2, which uses $(n - 1)$ in the denominator of Equation (4.4) instead of n, is often used in place of $\hat{\gamma}(0)$. The corresponding estimator of the autocorrelation is given by

$$\hat{\rho}(\tau) = \frac{\hat{\gamma}(\tau)}{\hat{\gamma}(0)} \tag{4.5}$$

Because it is assumed that the mean and the variance are stable, we estimate the variance using all the measurements.

Intuitively, it makes sense to use the autocovariance (or the autocorrelation) as a measure of the dependency between variables which are a specified number (τ) of time units apart, as may be realised from the following reasoning: We define high values as values that are higher than the mean, and low ones as values lower than the mean. If X_i and X_j are positively related, their values tend to be either both high or both low. In either case the corresponding product in the sum of Equation (4.4) will be positive. If they are negatively related, a high X_i value tends to be accompanied by a low X_j value and vice versa. In either case, the corresponding product in the above sum will be negative. If X_i and X_j are unrelated, positive and negative products will appear at random. Therefore, the above sum will be 0 or close to 0.

Example 4.1

We want to estimate the lag 1 and lag 2 autocovariance of the stationary sequence of random variables $\{X_1, X_2, X_3, X_4, X_5\}$ based on its realization $\{x_1, x_2, x_3, x_4, x_5\}$. The time series includes 5 consecutive values measured one day apart; the corresponding time axis includes the values 1 through 5 corresponding to the 5 days. x_1 is the value measured on day # 1, x_2 is the value measured on day # 2, ..., x_5 is the value measured on day # 5. To estimate the lag 1 autocovariance, we calculate

$$\frac{(x_1 - \overline{x})(x_2 - \overline{x}) + (x_2 - \overline{x})(x_3 - \overline{x}) + (x_3 - \overline{x})(x_4 - \overline{x}) + (x_4 - \overline{x})(x_5 - \overline{x})}{5 - 1}$$

The lag 2 autocovariance may be calculated using the same principle. We calculate

$$\frac{(x_1 - \overline{x})(x_3 - \overline{x}) + (x_2 - \overline{x})(x_4 - \overline{x}) + (x_3 - \overline{x})(x_5 - \overline{x})}{5 - 2}$$

As the lag increases, the number of pairs of values available to estimate the covariance declines (see Equation 4.4).

4.1.2 Stationary Time Series Models

We now introduce some simple stationary time series models for our future use.

4.1.2.1   White noise

The time series $X_1, X_2, \ldots, X_n, \ldots$ is called white noise if

1. X_i are identically distributed with zero mean and the same finite variance.
2. $\text{Cov}[X_i, X_j] = 0$ when $i \neq j$.

The autocorrelation function (ACF) is the autocorrelation coefficient depicted as a function of the lag. It follows from (2) above that the nonzero lag autocorrelations are all 0.

4.1.2.2   First order autoregressive (AR(1)) processes

The time series $X_1, X_2, \ldots, X_n, \ldots$ is called a first order autoregressive (AR(1)) process if

$$X_i - \mu = \phi(X_{i-1} - \mu) + a_i \qquad (4.6)$$

where ϕ is a constant and a_i are random variables from white noise. In (4.6), μ is the process mean. Equation (4.6) indicates the relationship between the term $(X_{i-1} - \mu)$, the deviation of the *previous* measurement from the mean and the deviation of the current measurement from the mean $(X_i - \mu)$. This models the dependency between the measurements. The magnitude of the dependency is determined by ϕ. This creates a positive dependency between the measurements when $\phi > 0$. When $|\phi| < 1$, the process is stationary. It may be shown that $\rho(\tau) = \phi^\tau$. There-fore, the ACF depicts a series of autocorrelation coefficients that are decaying exponentially as a function of the lag. When $\phi > 0$, we refer to this by saying that the process measurements are positively autocorre-lated. Conversely, when $\phi < 0$, we say the process measurements are negatively autocorrelated. And, in particular, when $\phi = 0$, $X_i = \mu + a_i$, i.e., the process is a mean plus white noise.

4.2   TESTS OF INDEPENDENCE OF MEASUREMENTS

For given time series data, we need to test whether the data are generated by statistically independent random variables or not. When the data follow a Gaussian distribution, this is equivalent to testing whether the autocorrelations of the random variables generating the data are 0 or not. It may be shown that if the stationary time series is not autocorrelated, then the sample autocorrelation for any lag larger than 0 follows a normal distribution with mean 0 and an approximate standard deviation $\frac{1}{\sqrt{n}}$ [1, p 32–4], where n is the length of the time series and large. This result is used to test whether a time series is autocorrelated or not.

Example 4.2

In clinical biochemistry, the quality of an assay, used to measure the concentration of creatinine, is monitored once a day by using the assay to measure the concentration of creatinine in the same stable quality-control material. The initial results are used to construct an X control chart. If the control chart values depict a process in statistical control, the assay is assumed to be stable. Future values are depicted on the control chart to verify that the analytical level remains stable.

Figure 4.1 shows 66 consecutive values, used for the quality control of the assay. The cyclical nature of the pattern of values indicates that they may be positively autocorrelated.

Figure 4.2 shows all pairs of consecutive values, i.e., x_t versus x_{t+1}.

The estimated lag 1 autocorrelation calculated using these pairs of consecutive values is 0.273. If the absolute value of the estimated autocorrelation is $> \frac{2}{\sqrt{66}} - 0.246$, the autocorrelation is statistically significantly different from 0 at the 5 % level of significance. Therefore, the series of creatinine values is significantly autocorrelated.

Figure 4.3 depicts the estimated autocorrelation function of the time series. It shows a 95 % confidence band for the autocorrelation function with limits of $\pm \frac{2}{\sqrt{n}}$ for each lag, assuming the time series is not

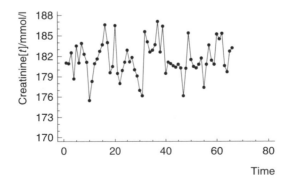

Figure 4.1 Quality control measurement values of a creatinine assay. The same stable quality-control material was used, and the results were depicted as a function of time (number of days) elapsed since the last calibration of the assay.

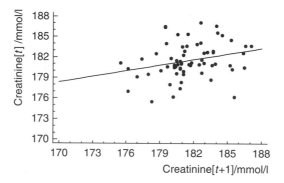

Figure 4.2 Scatter diagram of the results of the control measurements made of a creatinine assay at time t (y-axis) versus the result made at time $t + 1$ (one time unit ahead of it (x-axis)). The line depicts the regression of the former quantity on the latter.

autocorrelated. Therefore, if all the autocorrelations are within the dashed lines, we conclude that the sequence is not autocorrelated. In the present case, the lags 1, 6, 14, and 15 autocorrelations are significantly different from zero.

We need to point out that the sample autocorrelation function is based on the assumption that the underlying process is stationary. Namely, we assumed that the mean of the process is a constant. However, the ACF plot may falsely show significant autocorrelations if the underlying random process does not have a constant mean.

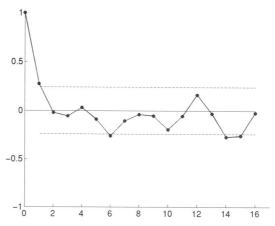

Figure 4.3 The autocorrelation function[a] with 95 % confidence interval limits[b] of 66 consecutive quality control measurements of a creatinine assay.
[a] The autocorrelation function is the autocorrelation coefficient as a function of its lag.
[b] The two dashed lines depict the upper, and the lower limit, respectively, of the 95% confidence intervals of the autocorrelation coefficients.

Example 4.3

Figure 4.4 shows 450 data points generated by three Gaussian distributions, each generating 150 consecutive values. All distributions had a variance of 1.0, while the mean was 0.0, 2.0, and 1.0, respectively, and all values were generated independent of each other. The time series generated was not stationary because the mean of the process was not kept constant.

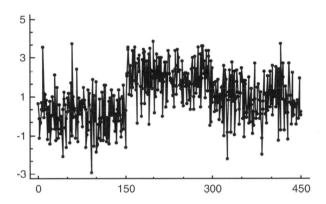

Figure 4.4 Four hundred and fifty statistically independent results generated by Gaussian distributions using simulation[a]. The x-axis depicts the sequence number of the values and the y-axis depicts the value generated.
[a] The mean value of the distribution generating the first 150 values was 0.0, that of the distribution generating the next 150 values was 2.0, and that of the distribution generating the last 150 values was 1.0. The standard deviation of all 3 distributions was 1.0.

Figure 4.5 shows the corresponding ACF plot with a 95 % confidence band for white noise.

This is the pattern that one would expect if the measurements were strongly autocorrelated. Therefore, using the ACF to check whether the process is autocorrelated may be misleading, unless the time series is stationary [2].

We recommend a 'runs test' to supplement the ACF plot. The runs test of randomness is a nonparametric test based on runs up and down. For a time series generated by $X_1, X_2, \ldots$ we form a sequence of $(n-1)$ plus and minus signs by noting the signs of successive differences generated by $D_i = X_{i+1} - X_i$ for $i = 1, 2, \ldots, n-1$. A run is defined as a succession of one or more identical signs that is preceded and followed by a different

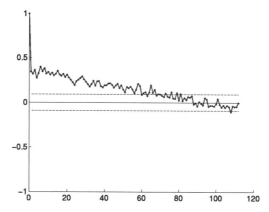

Figure 4.5 The autocorrelation function[a] with 95 % confidence interval limits[b] of 450 statistically independent values generated by Gaussian distributions[c] using simulation.
[a] The autocorrelation function is the autocorrelation coefficient as a function of its lag.
[b] The two dashed lines depict the upper, and the lower limit, respectively, of the 95 % confidence intervals of the autocorrelation coefficients.
[c] The mean value of the distribution generating the first 150 values was 0.0, that of the distribution generating the next 150 values was 2.0, and that of the distribution generating the last 150 values was 1.0. The standard deviation of all 3 distributions was 1.0.

sign or no sign at all. A run comprising positive signs is referred to as a 'run up' and one comprising negative signs, a 'run down'. For example, the sequence $\{1, 7, 3, 2, 5, 6\}$ is transformed to the difference sequence $\{6, -4, -1, 3, 1\}$ by calculating $7 - 1 = 6, 3 - 7 = -4$, etc. This series in turn is transformed to the sign sequence $\{+, -, -, +, +\}$. We denote the random variables corresponding to the numbers of up-runs and down-runs by R_u and R_d, respectively. In this example, $n = 6$, $R_u = 2$ (two sequences of plusses), and $R_d = 1$ (one sequence of minuses). The test statistic is the total number of runs, $V = R_u + R_d$. Here the value of V is 3. The null hypothesis is that the sequence $\{X_i, i = 1, \ldots, n\}$ is random. The distribution of V under the null hypothesis was derived and given in a table in Gibbons (1986) [3]. For large samples, the standard normal distribution can be used with

$$Z = \frac{V - (2n - 1)/3}{\sqrt{\dfrac{16n - 29}{90}}} \qquad (4.7)$$

where $\frac{2n-1}{3}$ is the approximate mean of V, and $\frac{16n-29}{90}$ the approximate variance. A continuity correction of ± 0.5 can be incorporated in the numerator of Z. In the above example, the approximate mean and variance of V are 3.67 and 0.74, respectively. For illustrative purposes we calculate the large sample test statistic with continuity correction. It is

$$Z = \frac{3 - 3.67 + 0.5}{\sqrt{0.74}} = -0.20.$$

Had the sample been large, the hypothesis, that the series is random, could not have been rejected at the $\alpha = 0.05$ significance level since the test statistic does not exceed (in absolute value) the cut off value of $\Phi^{-1}(1 - \frac{\alpha}{2}) = 1.96$, obtained from the standard Gaussian distribution. For the data plotted in Figure 4.4, the p-value $- 0.36$, indicating the data are not autocorrelated.

4.3 CONTROL CHARTS FOR AUTOCORRELATED DATA

In this section we first analyse the impact of autocorrelation on traditional control charts. Then we discuss two types of control charts that may be used in the presence of autocorrelated data.

4.3.1 Performance of Traditional Control Charts

Many statisticians and statistical process control (SPC) practitioners have found that autocorrelation in process data has impact on the performance of the traditional SPC charts. Autocorrelation may be caused by the measurement system, the dynamics of the process, or both. In many process industries, the data may exhibit a drifting behaviour. In biology, random biological variation, e.g., the random burst in the secretion of some substance that influences the blood pressure, may have a sustained effect so that several consecutive measurements are all influenced by the same random phenomenon. When the sampling interval is short, autocorrelation, especially positive autocorrelation of the data, is a concern. In the following example we study the impact of positive autocorrelation on the performance of various traditional control charts. To produce autocorrelated data we use simulation of the stationary first order autoregressive (AR(1)) process with $0 \leq \phi < 1$.

Example 4.4

The aim of the study was to assess the impact of various magnitudes of autocorrelation on the type-1 error rate expressed as the in-control ARL and on the type-2 error rate expressed as the out-of-control ARL for various changes in the process mean value. The magnitude of the auto-correlation was varied, by changing the value of ϕ of the AR(1) process (see Equation (4.6)). For each value of ϕ, the ARL was measured when the underlying process was in statistical control and when it was not. Simulation was used to study the impact of each type of time series. In each case, at least 2000 time series were generated. For a stable process (no change in process mean), the run length was measured for each series and the average value computed to obtain the in-control ARL. For an unstable process the mean value was changed during the simulation of a series and the run length then measured. The average of the 2000 series was calculated to obtain the out-of-control ARL. We studied the impact on the X chart, the CUSUM chart, and the EWMA chart. For the X chart, 3σ control limits were used. For the EWMA chart, λ was 0.2 and the control limits were also the 3σ limits. For the CUSUM chart we used the ARLs reported by Lucas [4]. The parameters used were, $h = 5.0$ and $k = 0.5$, for the tabular form of the chart. For reasons presented in Section 4.4, the sample standard deviation (see Equation (4.11)) was used in place of the estimate based on the moving range (see Equation (4.12)).

The results of the study are shown in Table 4.1. Column 1 shows the magnitude of the autocorrelation, ranging from no autocorrelation ($\phi = 0$) to $\phi = 0.9$. Column 2 shows, for each value of ϕ, the magnitudes of the mean value changes studied in the unit of process standard deviation (0.0, 0.5, 1.0, 2.0, and 3.0 standard deviation). Column 3 shows the behaviour of the X chart. The in-control ARL is not adversely affected by the presence of autocorrelation. When $\phi \leq 0.25$, the autocorrelation has small impact on the out-of-control ARL. When $\phi \geq 0.5$, however, the autocorrelation has a large impact on the ARL. The in-control ARL and the out-of-control ARL both increase when ϕ increases. The effects are especially clear when the mean shifts are small. In summary, when the autocorrelation is medium to large, the X chart will have difficulty in detecting small mean shifts. Columns 4 and 5 show the behaviour of the CUSUM and EWMA chart, respectively. When the process measurements are positively autocorrelated, even as weakly as $\phi = 0.25$, the in-control ARL is adversely affected. When $\phi = 0.25$, the in-control ARL for the CUSUM and EWMA charts are reduced to 119.35 and 139.55 from values of 465.00 and 547.71 when $\phi = 0$. Even in the presence of a weak autocorrelation, the charts will give frequent false alarms. On the other hand, the impact on the out-of-control ARLs of CUSUM and EWMA charts is relatively small. Therefore, when a process is positively autocorrelated, the in-control ARL of CUSUM and EWMA charts will be greatly affected, and false alarms will occur.

Table 4.1 Average run length (ARL) of X chart, cumulative sum (CUSUM) chart, and exponentially weighted moving average (EWMA) chart as a function of step changes of the process mean of increasing magnitudes (0.0 through 3.0 process standard deviation) and increasing positive autocorrelation of the data.

ϕ^a	Step change of process mean value	ARL (each value calculated from 2000 time series generated by simulation)		
		X chart ($k^b = 3.0$)	CUSUM chart ($h^c = 5.0$, $k^d = 0.5$)	EWMA chart ($\lambda^e = 0.2$, $L = 3.0$)
0.00	0.0	370.40	465.00	547.71
	0.5	155.21	38.00	44.60
	1.0	43.89	10.40	10.75
	2.0	6.30	4.01	3.73
	3.0	2.00	2.57	2.38
0.25	0.0	381.60	119.35	139.50
	0.5	160.53	30.02	32.81
	1.0	46.61	10.58	10.72
	2.0	7.25	4.16	3.85
	3.0	2.21	2.64	2.41
0.50	0.0	400.74	49.23	56.00
	0.5	181.15	25.76	26.96
	1.0	56.42	11.43	10.79
	2.0	9.16	4.34	4.00
	3.0	2.60	2.64	2.50
0.75	0.0	496.04	30.98	31.45
	0.5	235.98	22.74	21.82
	1.0	74.33	12.67	11.30
	2.0	14.42	4.73	4.56
	3.0	3.59	2.83	2.58
0.90	0.0	833.59	29.02	26.24
	0.5	413.03	24.40	21.09
	1.0	157.72	15.38	13.19
	2.0	27.09	5.84	5.08
	3.0	6.24	2.85	2.72

[a] ϕ is the parameter of the autoregressive function of first order (AR(1)) that generated the data used. It was varied as shown in column 1. The larger ϕ is, the more autocorrelated the generated data are. For each combination of ϕ value and step change of the process mean (column 2), 2000 time series were generated using simulation. The white noise of the AR(1) was simulated using a Gaussian distribution with variance 1.0 and mean equal to 0.0.

[b] The number of sample standard deviations that the control limits are removed from the centreline.

[c] Control limit in the unit of process standard deviation.

[d] $k = \frac{\mu_1 - \mu_0}{2\sigma}$. Therefore, $k = 0.5$ implies that μ_1 is 1σ larger than μ_0, i.e., that the chart is designed to detect a change in the process mean of 1σ.

[e] The weight parameter of the EWMA statistic.

We only report the results for positively autocorrelated series since positive autocorrelation is by far the most predominant type within biology. For a study of the impact of negative autocorrelation, the reader is referred to Zhang (2000) [5]. We only considered a step mean change, where the mean changes instantaneously and then remains stable at the new level. However, other types of changes are possible, such as the exponential shift (see the discussion in Harris and Ross (1991) [6]).

4.3.2 The Residual Chart

To accommodate autocorrelated data, various SPC methodologies have been developed during recent years. One approach, proposed by Alwan and Roberts (1988) [7], is to use a process residual chart. This procedure requires one to model the process data. For example, an AR(1) model is identified and the parameter ϕ is estimated from the data. Using this estimate and the sample mean, the value predicted from the AR(1) function is calculated and subtracted from the observed value to obtain the process residual (see Chapter 5). Assuming the model is correct, the residuals are statistically uncorrelated to each other. Therefore, traditional SPC charts such as the X chart, the CUSUM chart (e.g., Runger, Willemain, and Prabhu (1995) [8]), and the EWMA chart (Lu and Reynolds (1999) [9]) may be applied to the residuals. Once a change of the mean or variance of the residual process is detected, it is concluded that the mean or variance of the process itself has changed. It is assumed that the in-control process is stationary.

The residual chart has the advantage that it can be applied to any autocorrelated time series, in some cases even if the data are from a nonstationary process. However, the X residual chart, which is an X chart applied to the residuals, does not have the same properties as the ordinary X chart, even though the residuals for a true model are statistically uncorrelated. It has been shown that sometimes the detection capability of an X residual chart is poor for a small mean shift [10]. The CUSUM residual and EWMA residual charts in general perform much better than the X residual chart. However, all the residual charts require time series modelling, which is a big disadvantage.

4.3.3 Traditional Control Charts with Adjusted Control Limits

Another more direct approach is to modify the existing SPC charts by adjusting the control limits. For example, Vasilopoulos and Stamboulis

[11] proposed the $\overline{X}$ chart with modified limits to monitor autocorrelated data. Their studies, however, were limited to some specific time series models, e.g., the AR(1).

Here we will introduce the EWMA stationary (EWMAST) chart proposed by Zhang [12]. The chart is simple to implement, and no time series modelling effort is required. It is constructed by charting the EWMA statistic defined in Equation (3.11). However, instead of the variance given in Equation (3.13), which applies for a stationary process without autocorrelation, the variance for the EWMA statistic Z_i is derived under the assumption that the process is autocorrelated and stationary. At each point in time, say i time units subsequent to the start of the time series, Zhang [12] derived the variance of the EWMA from the process variance when the process is stationary without autocorrelation (see Equation (3.13)) by an adjustment using the following term

$$2 \sum_{k=1}^{i-1} \rho(k)(1-\lambda)^k [1 - (1-\lambda)^{2(i-k)}] \tag{4.8}$$

where i is the time unit number and k is the lag of the autocorrelation (the term includes $(i-1)$ autocorrelations). Thus, the variance of the EWMA is inflated if the process is positively autocorrelated, deflated if the process is negatively autocorrelated, and unchanged if the process is not autocorrelated. The following equation is used to calculate the variance adjusted for autocorrelation

$$\sigma_{Z_i}^2 = \left(\frac{\lambda}{2-\lambda}\right)\sigma^2 \left[1 - (1-\lambda)^{2i} + 2\sum_{k=1}^{i-1} \rho(k)(1-\lambda)^k [1 - (1-\lambda)^{2(i-k)}]\right] \tag{4.9}$$

When i is large, the variance in the above can be approximated by

$$\sigma_Z^2 = \left(\frac{\lambda}{2-\lambda}\right)\sigma^2 \left[1 + 2\sum_{k=1}^{M} \rho(k)(1-\lambda)^k [1 - (1-\lambda)^{2(M-k)}]\right] \tag{4.10}$$

for $i > M$ where $M \geq 25$. Thus, all autocorrelation coefficients of lag equal to or larger than M are ignored. The ACF usually has to be estimated from the data and 75 observations at least are required to estimate a coefficient. It follows that at least 100 observations are needed before the above equation may be used. The EWMAST chart is constructed in the same

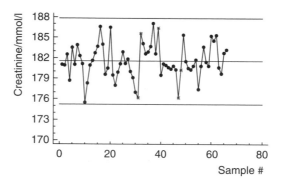

Figure 4.6 *X* chart calculated using 66 consecutive creatinine assay quality-control measurement values. The values are depicted on the chart.

way as the EWMA chart except that the adjusted variance is used to obtain the theoretically proper control limits.

Example 4.5

In Example 4.2 we examined a time series of creatinine values that was positively autocorrelated, but weakly so.

Figure 4.6 shows an *X* chart constructed from these data and with the values depicted on the chart. All values are within the control limits. However, there are certain indications that the process is not in control

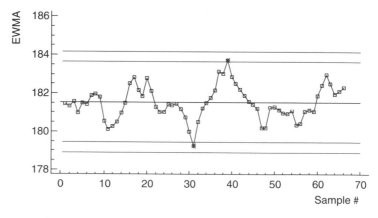

Figure 4.7 The exponentially weighted moving average (EWMA) calculated using the values of 66 consecutive creatinine assay quality-control measurement values. $\lambda = 0.2$. Control limits that are 3 sample standard deviations removed from the centreline are shown. The outer, but not the inner, control limits are adjusted for the autocorrelation of the values. The UCL and LCL of the EWMA chart are based on (3.18) and (3.19). The UCL and LCL of the EWMAST chart are based on (4.10).

as evidenced by the starred data points signifying either a run of 8 or more values on the same side of the mean or two out of three consecutive values outside the 2 standard deviation warning limit or both.

Figure 4.7 depicts the EWMA with traditional control limits and the EWMAST limits adjusted for autocorrelation. Two values are outside the traditional control limits. These outliers are probably caused by the positive autocorrelation. This is supported by the fact that all values are within the EWMAST control limits.

4.4   EFFECT OF CHOICE OF PROCESS STANDARD DEVIATION ESTIMATOR

In Sections 4.3.1 to 4.3.3, we have shown that autocorrelation impacts on the performance of the traditional SPC charts and discussed the use of alternative charts. To complicate matters it appears that the choice of process standard deviation estimator affects the behaviour of the control charts in the presence of autocorrelation.

When the data are from a stationary process, as in Example 4.4 and the study in [5], the process sample standard deviation,

$$S = \sqrt{\frac{\sum_{i=1}^{k} (X_i - \overline{X})^2}{k - 1}} \tag{4.11}$$

where k is the number of samples, was used to estimate the process standard deviation as discussed in Section 4.1.1. For the residual chart in Section 4.3.2, the process sample standard deviation or the estimators based on the white noise standard deviation, which are based on time series modelling, were used in the literature. For the EWMAST chart proposed in [12], the process sample standard deviation was used. In the study by Zhang [13], comparisons of the estimators of the process variance were made using the minimum mean squared error (MSE) criterion. In general the process sample variance was found to be a better estimator than that based on the process modelling.

When the measurements are independent and follow a Gaussian distribution,

$$\hat{\sigma}_{MR} = \sum_{j=2}^{k} \frac{|X_j - X_{j-1}|}{d_2(k - 1)} \tag{4.12}$$

where k is the number of samples and the constant $d_2 = 1.128$ is an unbiased estimator of σ, i.e., $E[\hat{\sigma}_{MR}] = \sigma$. Since this estimate is little influenced by variation due to assignable causes [14], it was chosen in favour of the estimate given in Equation (4.11) when estimating the process standard deviation for the X chart. However, when the process is autocorrelated, $\hat{\sigma}_{MR}$ may not be unbiased and thus may not be a good estimator of the process standard deviation. In Appendix C, it is shown that when the process is an AR(1) process with parameter ϕ,

$$E[\hat{\sigma}_{MR}] = \sigma\sqrt{1 - \phi} \qquad (4.13)$$

Thus, in this case the process standard deviation estimator $\hat{\sigma}_{MR}$ is a biased estimator of the process standard deviation, and the bias is a function of ϕ. If $\hat{\sigma}_{MR}$ is used to estimate σ and construct the control limits for the X chart or EWMAST chart (see Equation (4.10)) when $\phi > 0$, both the in-control and the out-of-control ARL will be smaller than when the sample standard deviation is used. Thus, when the process is in control, more false alarms will be generated. Conversely, from Equation (4.13) when the process is negatively autocorrelated, i.e., $\phi < 0$, on average $\hat{\sigma}_{MR}$ will be larger than the true process standard deviation. In this case, when the process is out of control, the out-of-control alarms will be delayed. Similar to [13], we performed a simulation to compare the performance of $\hat{\sigma}_{MR}$ and the sample standard deviation S given in Equation (4.11) using the criterion of the minimum mean squared error. From the simulation, we conclude that the sample standard deviation is a much better estimator than the moving ranges. We propose the use of the process sample standard deviation in Equation (4.11) to construct the control limits for the X chart and EWMAST chart in the presence of autocorrelation and stationarity.

However, one must be sure that the process is really stationary. If a process is not autocorrelated, but does not have a constant mean, the test given in Equation (4.7) may reveal the property of randomness. However, if a process is autocorrelated with an unstable mean we may miss the fact that it is nonstationary if we use the EWMAST chart because this chart is based on the assumption that the process is stationary. Thus, there may be situations where it is relevant to test if a process is stationary or nonstationary. Such tests are reviewed, e.g., in Box *et al.* [1, p 207–11].

REFERENCES

[1] Box GEP, Jenkins GM, and Reinsel GC. Time Series Analysis: Forecasting and Control. 3rd edition, Prentice Hall, New Jersey, 1994.

[2] Winkel P, and Zhang NF. Effects of uncertainty components such as recalibration on the performance of quality control charts. Scand J Clin Lab Invest 2005; 65:707–20.

[3] Gibbons JD. Encyclopedia of Statistical Sciences. 7: 555–62. Wiley and Sons Inc, New York, 1986.

[4] Lucas JM. The design and use of V-mask control schemes. J Qual Technol 1976; 8: 1–12.

[5] Zhang NF. Statistical control charts for monitoring the mean of a stationary process. J Stat Comput Sim 2000; 66:249–58.

[6] Harris TJ, and Ross WH. Statistical process control procedures for correlated observations. Can J Chem Eng 1991; 69:48–57.

[7] Alwan LC, and Roberts HV. Time series modelling for statistical process control. J Bus Econ Stat 1988; 6:87–95.

[8] Runger GC, Willemain TR, and Prabhu S. Average run lengths for CUSUM control charts applied to residuals. Commun Stat – Theor M 1995; 24:273–82.

[9] Lu CW, and Reynolds MR. EWMA control charts for monitoring the mean of autocorrelated processes. J Qual Technol 1999; 31:166–88.

[10] Zhang NF. Detection capability of residual control chart for stationary process data. J Appl Stat 1997; 24:475–92.

[11] Vasilopoulos AV, and Stamboulis AP. Modification of control chart limits in the presence of data correlation. J Qual Technol 1978; 1:20–30.

[12] Zhang NF. A statistical control chart for stationary process data. Technometrics 1998; 40:24–8.

[13] Zhang NF. Estimation of process variance in using SPC charts for a stationary process. Proceedings of Section of Physical and Engineering Sciences of the American Statistical Association 2002; 395:1–4.

[14] Duncan AJ. Quality Control and Industrial Statistics. McGraw-Hill, USA, 1986.

Part II

Risk Adjustment

5

Tools for Risk Adjustment

When outcome measures are compared between healthcare units, it is essential that the patients treated in the various units are comparable in terms of severity of disease, co-morbidity, and other factors that may influence the outcome. Otherwise, differences in case mix cannot be distinguished from differences in quality of care. Full comparability may be obtained experimentally, using random assignment of patients to the healthcare units.

If this approach is not taken, the case mix may differ between healthcare units. One may then attempt to compensate for these differences by using risk adjustment of the observational data [1]. Risk adjustment is based on various statistical techniques. In this chapter, we will review the techniques used. In subsequent chapters, we will explain how they may be applied for risk adjustment. It seems prudent to stress at the start that even if one uses all available statistical tools invented so far, full risk adjustment may not be possible. We have no assurance that our attempt to compensate for case-mix differences is going to work.

5.1 VARIABLES

The term variable is used to denote anything within a data set that varies. The techniques used in risk-adjustment are mainly linear regression techniques. Using these techniques a dependent variable is expressed as a linear function of one or more independent variables (or predictors or covariates) plus error. The independent variables are the risk factors or indicators of 'intervention', e.g., patient assignment to a specified

Statistical Development of Quality in Medicine   P. Winkel and N. F. Zhang
© 2007 John Wiley & Sons, Ltd

healthcare provider. The dependent variables are the outcome measures. An outcome measure is a variable, representing the outcomes of patient treatment and care. Variables may also be classified mathematically according to the type of data they represent (variable types). In the following, we will first describe the major mathematical types of variables. Then, we will discuss a clinical category of variables, namely outcome measures.

5.1.1   Mathematical Types of Variables

Variables may represent categorical or numerical data. Data used to allocate a patient to a specified category, such as male sex, are categorical data. Categorical data are binomial or binary if there are two possible categories, and multinomial if there are more than two. A variable representing multinomial data, say k categories ($k > 2$), is usually transformed into ($k - 1$) binary variables, each referring to a specified category where k is the number of possible categories. The remaining category is the reference category. Each of the binary variables is usually set equal to 1 if the patient belongs to the specified category and 0 otherwise. As an example, let us take an outcome variable. Say patients are classified into three types according to the result of an operation: (1) the patient died, (2) the patient had a nonfatal cardiac incident, or (3) the patient neither died nor had a nonfatal cardiac incident. We arbitrarily define one of the three categories as the reference category. For instance, we may choose the category neither death nor nonfatal cardiac incident as the reference category. The variable *death* is 1 if the patient dies and 0 otherwise. The variable *cardiac incident* is 1 if the patient has a nonfatal cardiac incident and 0 otherwise. If the patient survives and does not have a nonfatal cardiac incident, both of the above two variables are 0. Categories may be nominal (they cannot be ordered meaningfully according to size) or ordinal (they can be ordered according to size). An example of the first type is blood group, and an example of the second type is cancer staging.

If the observations can only take numerical values, the resulting data are numerical. If they can only take up to a finite or a countable, infinite number of possible values, the data are discrete; otherwise they are continuous. The corresponding variables are referred to as discrete and continuous variables. Numerical data may meaningfully be subtracted from each other and multiplied. This is not so for ordinal categorical data (cancer stage 3 minus cancer stage 1 cannot meaningfully be equated with cancer stage 2).

5.1.2   Outcome Measures

An outcome measure may be continuous, like the length of stay in hospital, a satisfaction score, etc. A continuous outcome measure may be used directly as a dependent variable. Often the outcome of interest is an event, e.g., the death following admission to a hospital of a patient suffering from acute myocardial infarct (AMI). The event definition may include a time constraint, e.g., death during the first 30 days following admission, or it may not. In the former case, the outcome measure is a binary categorical variable (death, yes or no?). In the latter case, the outcome measure is continuous, i.e., the time until the event occurs. However, when the study is terminated, the time until the event, for instance death, is unknown for those patients who are still alive (their 'survival times' are censored), and this calls for a special type of analysis (see, e.g., [2]–[6]) that is not presented in this book. Another possibility is that the outcome is one of a number of distinct, mutually exclusive, and exhaustive events. For example the events may be death, nonfatal cardiac incident, or neither of these in diabetic patients during the first 30 days after a major operation. In this case, the outcome measure is a multinomial categorical variable. The outcome may also include multiple events, like the number of complications occurring in a patient during and/or following an operation, deaths per year, etc. In this case, the outcome measure is a discrete variable since it can only take integer values (in principle, an infinite number of integer values). However, they are countable as opposed to real numbers that are not countable.

Here we will review the analysis of continuous outcome measures (without censoring) and binary categorical outcome measures because they are the most commonly used outcome measures in clinical quality assurance and development.

5.2   STATISTICAL MODELS

Some kind of model is needed to transform the values of the independent variables and the dependent variable, into a regression equation, relating the former to the latter. Such a model describes the assumed relationship in mathematical terms and is based on assumptions. Ideally, the assumptions should be fulfilled for the model to produce reliable results. Therefore, these assumptions ought to be given some consideration. They should, a priori, appear reasonably realistic. If possible, they should be tested. In particular, if the model is known to be sensitive to deviations.

It may be advantageous to reflect upon the general structure of the system that one wants to analyse before a choice of model is made. Ideally, a model should be rich enough to mirror a general structure. The healthcare system may be viewed as a hierarchy of subsystems of units. At the lowest level, we have the patients (not literally, of course). They may be grouped into various clinical entities, for example patients suffering from diabetes, patients suffering from arthritis, patients suffering from acute myocardial infarction (AMI), etc. The second level may, for instance, be the physicians. Physicians may be grouped according to specialty, experience, etc. The third level is physician practices and/or hospital departments. They may be grouped according to volume, educational status, financial support, etc. A fourth level may be regions or countries. However, in reality the structure may not be that simple. For instance, the same physician may operate at more than one hospital, etc. Usually the outcomes of patients from a specified clinical entity are compared across the units of a higher level. For instance, the satisfaction scores of diabetic patients may be compared between physicians within a specified hospital. Or, in a slightly more complex version, the patient scores may be compared across physicians as well as across hospitals. In the latter example, the patients (the primary units) are sampled from each physician, the physicians (the secondary units) are sampled from each hospital, and the hospitals (the tertiary units) are sampled from say a geographical region.

In Section 5.3, we present regression models that may be applied when the outcome measure is continuous, and in Section 5.4 we present models that may be applied when the outcome measure is a binary variable. When the analysis is confined to a single group of patients, e.g., patients treated by the same physician, single level regression analysis should be applied. If several groups of patients are analysed, e.g., patients from three different hospitals, hierarchical linear regression should be used.

5.3 REGRESSION ON CONTINUOUS
OUTCOME MEASURES

Here we review the linear regression models for continuous outcome data. In Section 5.3.1 we present the single level linear regression. In this model there is no hierarchical structure. Only one level is represented, the patient level. In the subsequent two sections two important concepts are explained, residual variation and interaction. As a rule, a regression equation does not explain all the variation of the dependent variable.

This residual variation should be measured. How this may be done is explained in Section 5.3.2. The independent variables may influence each other in the sense that the relationship between one independent variable and the dependent outcome variable may depend on the value of a second independent variable. This phenomenon is referred to as interaction and is explained in Section 5.3.3. In Section 5.3.4 we address the situation where the data structure is hierarchical and hierarchical models usually should be applied.

5.3.1 Single Level Linear Regression

Regression may include one independent variable (simple regression) or several independent variables (multiple regression). The following invented example, relating duration of a surgical procedure to the operator's experience, illustrates the principles of simple regression.

Example 5.1

Table 5.1 shows the operating times of the first five operations performed by the same surgeon, using a new surgical procedure. We want to study

Table 5.1 Linear regression and power law regression of operation sequence # on duration of the operation.

Sequence # (x)	Operating time/hour (y)	Squared difference from mean $(y - 1.700)^2$	Linear[a] prediction $(\hat{y})$	Square of linear regression error $(y - \hat{y})^2$	Power law[b] prediction $(\hat{y})$	Square of power law error $(y - \hat{y})^2$
1	5.000	10.890	3.700	1.690	4.696	0.092
2	1.500	0.040	2.700	1.440	1.679	0.032
3	1.000	0.490	1.700	0.490	0.920	0.006
4	0.500	1.440	0.700	0.040	0.600	0.010
5	0.500	1.440	0.300	0.640	0.431	0.005
Sum	ND[c]	$TSS(adj)^d$ =14.300	ND[c]	SSE^e = 4.300	ND[c]	0.145

[a]Linear regression: operating time $= 4.7 - 1.0 \cdot$ sequence #.
[b]Power law: operating time $= 4.696$ sequence #$^{-1.484}$.
[c]Not determined.
[d]Total sum of squares, adjusted (adj).
[e]Sum of squares of errors.

the relationship between the skills of the operator (the dependent variable), expressed as the speed with which he/she finishes the procedure; and his/her experience (the independent variable), expressed as the sequence number of the procedure performed by him/her. To describe the relationship, a linear function may be tried. This type of function is characterised by two parameters: a, the intersection with the y-axis and b, the slope. We have

$$\text{operating time} = a + b \cdot \text{sequence\#} \qquad (5.1)$$

The problem is to find appropriate values for a and b. Assume that we have chosen $a = 5.0$ hour and $b = -1.0$ hour/sequence #. For each observation, we may calculate the value, predicted from this linear function. For example, for sequence # = 3.0, we have operating time $= 5.0 - 1.0 \cdot 3.0 = 2.0$ hour. To measure how good this prediction is, we calculate the error (also called the residual), which is defined as the difference between the observed and the predicted value. If it were zero, we would have a perfect fit between model and observation. In the example it is $1.0 - 2.0 = -1.0$ hour. In geometrical terms, this is the vertical distance from the observation to the chosen linear function (see Figure 5.1).

The square of the error is $(-1)^2 = 1$. To assess how well a given function fits the observations, we calculate the square of each error and add the results to obtain the sum of the squared errors (SSE). This is a measure of the deviations of the observations from the regression line. When a linear regression analysis is performed, the values of a and b that minimise this sum are found. In the example, the resulting values are

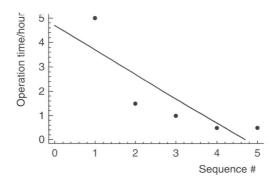

Figure 5.1   Linear regression of sequence # of operation on operation time/hour.

$a = 4.7$ hour and $b = -1.0$ hour/sequence #. The corresponding value of *SSE* is 4.3.

The assumption of a linear regression is that the relationship between the independent and the dependent variable is linear, except for random variation. Therefore, before doing a linear regression, one needs to assess the validity of this assumption. Figure 5.1 depicts the observed values of Example 5.1 and the linear regression line that we have just determined. The observations do not appear to be linearly related to the sequence #. Sometimes, a problem like this may be solved, by using some kind of transformation of the values of the independent variable or the values of the dependent one, or both. If the relationship between the variables after the transformation appears to be reasonably linear, the regression is carried out, using the transformed values. The result may be transformed back to the original metric, using the reverse transformation. We will try this approach using the data of Example 5.1.

Example 5.2

It turns out that a logarithmic transformation of both variables solves the linearity problem. Therefore, we transform the data of Example 5.1, by taking the logarithm of the values. We now need to find the values of a and b that minimise the *SSE* of the following relationship

$$\log(\text{operating time/hour}) = a + b \cdot \log(\text{sequence \#}) \qquad (5.2)$$

Figure 5.2 shows the relationship found, using linear regression. We have $a = 1.547$ and $b = -1.484$. This relationship seems to be linear except for random variation because the observed values scatter at random around the regression line.

Having transformed the problem into a linear problem and solved it, we need to transform the solution back to the original metric. By definition, we have $e^{\log(x)} = x$. To go back from the logarithmic coordinate system to the original one, we have to calculate the exponential function of the result. Therefore, we calculate

$$e^{\log(\text{operating time/hour})} = e^{(a+b \cdot \log(\text{sequence \#}))}, \text{implying}$$

$$\text{operating time/hour} = e^{1.547}(\text{sequence \#})^{-1.484}$$

$$= 4.696(\text{sequence \#})^{-1.484}.$$

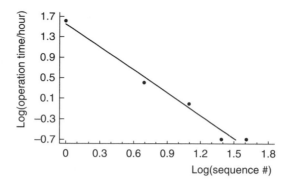

Figure 5.2 Linear regression of the logarithm (log) of sequence # of operation on log(operation time/hour).

This type of function ($Y = bX^c$) is called the power law. Using the power law, the predicted values and *SSE* may be calculated. For example, for sequence # = 3.0, we obtain the predicted value, $4.696 \cdot 3.0^{-1.484} = 0.920$, the error $0.920 - 1.000 = -0.080$, and the squared error 0.0064.

It is the rule, rather than the exception, in clinical work, that there is more than one independent variable. In this situation multiple linear regression should be used. The problem in multiple linear regressions is to find a linear function of the following type

$$Y_i = a + b_1 X_{1i} + b_2 X_{2i} + b_3 X_{3i} + \cdots + b_p X_{pi} \qquad (5.3)$$

where Y_i is the *i*th observation of the dependent variable, X_{1i}, X_{2i}, etc are the *p* independent variables as measured in patient # *i*, and a, b_1, b_2, etc are the constant and the coefficients of the function, determined by using the principle explained above, i.e., the constant and the coefficients are determined so that the sum of squared errors *SSE* becomes as small as possible. Statistically, it is assumed that the data may be described, using the following model

$$Y_i = \alpha + \beta_1 X_{1i} + \beta_2 X_{2i} + \beta_3 X_{3i} + \cdots + \beta_p X_{pi} + \varepsilon_i \qquad (5.4)$$

where ε_i is a random deviation from the value of the unknown linear function, the parameters of which we want to estimate. It is often assumed to follow a Gaussian distribution with expected value 0 and standard deviation σ, ε_i and are assumed to be statistically independent.

Because the parameters of the linear function and σ are actually unknown, they have to be estimated from the observations. It turns out that the constant and coefficients (see Equation (5.3)) that we determined by minimising the SSE are the best estimates. The same reasoning, of course, applies to simple regression.

Once the best linear function is estimated, one may calculate for each value of the dependent variable the corresponding (predicted) value, using the estimated function and the values of the independent variables (just as in the above example). The difference between observed and predicted value is the error or residual. For each independent variable, the linearity assumption may be examined, as shown in the above examples. Various analyses of the residuals may be conducted. Ideally, they should follow a Gaussian distribution and be independent of each other. A careful study of the residuals of a model is important to validate the linear model used and to detect unusual observations (outliers). For details, the reader is referred to statistical textbooks (see, e.g., [6]).

Example 5.3

Wetterslev et al. [7] studied the effect of optimising pulmonary compliance with peroperative application of a positive end expiratory pressure (PEEP) on postoperative complications and arterial oxygen tension on day 2 (a-PO2-day-2), following upper abdominal surgery. Forty patients were randomised to either PEEP or no PEEP. Arterial oxygen tension during the operation (a-PO2), the duration of the operation (op-time), the preoperative functional residual capacity (FRC) reduction in 30° head tilt-down position (ΔFRC), and smoking status, expressed as number of cigarette pack year (pack-year) were measured in each patient as were other clinical and demographic data.

Table 5.2 presents the data. There are two dependent variables, a continuous one (a-PO2-day-2) and a binary one (Cpl, 1 if complication is present, otherwise 0). Here, we will study the continuous one. The independent variables include four continuous ones (a-PO2, ΔFRC, op-time, and pack-year) and one binary (PEEP, 1 if PEEP was applied and 0 otherwise). The four continuous independent variables may be considered risk factors. The problem is to adjust for the influence of these risk factors and then assess the impact of the intervention (PEEP) on the dependent variable (a-PO2-day-2). This may be achieved, using multiple

Table 5.2 Independent and dependent variables from study by Wetterslev *et al.* [7].

i	a-PO2$_i$	ΔFRC$_i$	op-time$_i$	pack-year$_i$	PEEP$_i$	a-PO2-day-2$_i$	Cpl$_i$	$\hat{p}_i^c$	$\hat{p}_i^2$
		Independent variables^a				Dependent variables^b			
1	18.49	2.69	140	10	1	11.10	0	0.0031	0.000010
2	14.63	2.95	290	0	1	9.20	0	0.0034	0.000011
3	19.45	2.54	165	10	0	11.00	0	0.0059	0.000035
4	14.83	1.77	210	3	0	7.90	0	0.0281	0.000787
5	24.92	2.40	270	14	0	9.70	0	0.0374	0.001401
6	14.97	2.35	353	5	1	6.90	0	0.0428	0.001828
7	15.58	0.66	55	0	0	7.00	0	0.0481	0.002310
8	17.25	2.25	180	24	1	9.00	0	0.0521	0.002718
9	17.75	1.41	180	5	0	8.20	0	0.0550	0.003025
10	16.50	1.92	310	4	1	8.99	0	0.0637	0.004062
11	24.85	2.58	400	10	1	8.70	0	0.0676	0.004570
12	26.67	1.37	260	1	1	10.90	0	0.0951	0.009048
13	21.82	1.13	208	3	0	10.10	0	0.1106	0.012238
14	17.70	1.58	195	16	1	8.90	0	0.1216	0.014777
15	18.67	1.30	235	8	1	9.70	1	0.1568	0.024585
16	23.63	1.37	330	1	0	7.90	1	0.1857	0.034474
17	8.98	0.52	180	0	1	8.40	1	0.2177	0.047397
18	14.31	1.50	180	24	0	9.10	0	0.2382	0.056746
19	20.54	0.99	320	0	1	10.50	0	0.3059	0.093549
20	13.92	1.38	95	35	0	7.60	1	0.3251	0.105690
21	9.20	0.36	230	0	1	7.50	0	0.4121	0.169828
22	19.93	0.77	210	12	0	9.40	0	0.4175	0.174347
23	14.59	0.59	285	0	0	5.50	0	0.4305	0.185320
24	10.41	0.49	270	0	1	7.20	0	0.4467	0.199530
25	14.09	0.90	112	28	1	9.90	1	0.4684	0.219416
26	16.37	0.98	295	11	0	7.80	0	0.5053	0.255349
27	16.53	1.62	325	24	0	9.10	0	0.5407	0.292398
28	15.47	2.09	290	40	1	8.70	0	0.5692	0.324021
29	13.80	2.95	585	30	0	8.50	1	0.6351	0.403391
30	18.43	1.26	200	36	0	7.70	0	0.6918	0.478575
31	21.00	1.31	365	20	1	7.20	1	0.7163	0.513082
32	19.65	0.27	245	10	1	9.30	1	0.7338	0.538436
33	13.89	0.78	325	15	0	5.80	1	0.7711	0.594566
34	13.43	1.29	420	20	0	missing	1	0.8293	0.687785
35	18.55	1.18	225	40	0	8.50	1	0.8413	0.707867
36	11.07	1.35	470	25	1	7.10	1	0.9236	0.853033
37	22.04	0.36	450	10	0	7.50	1	0.9558	0.913478
38	14.05	0.50	343	27	1	6.90	1	0.9629	0.927153
39	11.15	0.84	285	52	1	7.70	1	0.9868	0.973754
40	7.61	0.06	350	45	0	5.70	1	0.9979	0.995719

Sum of squared probabilities   10.82800

^{a} The independent variables are, arterial oxygen tension during operation (a-PO2$_i$), pre-operative functional residual capacity reduction (ΔFRC$_i$), operating time/minute (op-time$_i$), cigarette smoking in pack-year (pack-year$_i$), and peroperative application of end expiratory pressure (PEEP$_i$).

^{b} The dependent variables are, arterial oxygen tension on day 2 following operation (a-PO2-day-2$_i$) and presence of postoperative complication (Cpl$_i$).

^{c} Estimated probability of postoperative complication in patient # i based on regression of a-PO2$_i$, ΔFRC$_i$, op-time$_i$, pack-year$_i$, and PEEP$_i$ on logit(p_i) where p_i is probability of postoperative complication.

Table 5.3 Output from regression of arterial oxygen tension during operation (a-$PO2_i$), pre-operative functional residual capacity reduction (ΔFRC_i), operating time/minute (op-time), and peroperative application of end expiratory pressure ($PEEP_i$) on arterial oxygen tension on day 2 following operation (a-PO2-day-2_i).

Parameter[a]	Estimate	Standard error of estimate	p
α	6.090	0.763	0.000
β_1	0.144	0.038	0.001
β_2	0.620	0.217	0.007
β_3	−0.005	0.002	0.003
β_4	0.699	0.322	0.037

[a] Parameters of the regression: $Y_i = \alpha + \beta_1 \cdot \text{a-PO2}_i + \beta_2 \cdot \Delta FRC_i + \beta_3 \cdot \text{op-time}_i + \beta_4 PEEP_i + \varepsilon_i$.

regression of a-PO2, ΔFRC, op-time, pack-year, and PEEP on a-PO2-day-2. Pack-year did not contribute significantly to the prediction and was, therefore, excluded from further analyses.

Table 5.3 shows part of the output from a program that calculated the regression of a-PO2, ΔFRC, op-time, and PEEP on a-PO2-day-2. The estimates of the constant α and the coefficients (β_1, β_2, β_3, and β_4) are shown in column 2.

The coefficient of an independent variable X is equal to the change of the dependent variable if all other independent variables are kept constant and the value of X changes by one unit. Therefore, the effect of each independent variable may be assessed when adjusted for that of the other independent variables. The standard deviations of the estimates (standard errors) are shown in column 3. In column 4, the p-values calculated by the program are shown. The coefficient of PEEP is significantly different from zero ($p < 0.05$). Therefore, we may conclude that PEEP has an effect on a-PO2-day-2, in addition to the effect of the risk factors. The regression equation is as follows

$$\text{a-PO2-day-2} = 6.090 + 0.144\,\text{a-PO2} + 0.620\Delta\text{FRC}$$
$$- 0.005\,\text{op-time} + 0.699\,\text{PEEP} \qquad (5.5)$$

The estimated effect of a positive end expiratory pressure (PEEP = 1) on a-PO2-day-2 is 0.7 kPa.

In clinical problems, there are often several independent variables (say 20 or even more) that are potentially related to the dependent variable. In this case, it may be desirable to remove variables that are redundant. A redundant variable does not contribute significantly (either at the $p = 0.01$ or $p = 0.05$ level of significance) to the prediction when the essential variables have been included in the regression equation. There are various techniques that may be used, and they do not always lead to the same conclusion. Redundant variables may either be removed automatically by a statistical program or semi automatically by the combined use of statistical programs and clinical reasoning. The interested reader is referred to [6, 8, 9, 10, 11, 12].

Example 5.4

In Table 5.2 the data of the 40 patients are shown. We will use Equation (5.5) to predict the a-PO2-day-2 of the first patient who received the PEEP intervention. Inserting his/her values in the equation, we obtain

$$\text{a-PO2-day-2} = 6.090 + 0.144 \, \text{a-PO2} + 0.620 \, \Delta\text{FRC} - 0.005 \, \text{op-time}$$
$$+ 0.699 \, \text{PEEP} = 6.090 + 0.144 \cdot 18.49 + 0.620 \cdot 2.69$$
$$- 0.005 \cdot 140 + 0.699 \cdot 1 = 10.42 \, \text{kPa}.$$

The observed value was 11.10 kPa. Therefore, the error is $11.10 - 10.42 = 1.74 \, \text{kPa}$.

In the above example, we modelled the risk factors and the treatment using a fixed-effect model. When one is comparing the quality of treatment between healthcare providers, e.g., two different hospitals, an approach similar to that of the above example may be taken. One defines a categorical variable, HOSPITAL-1 that is equal to 1 if the patient was treated at hospital number one, and 0 otherwise. If there are more than two hospitals, say k, one would define $k - 1$ binary variables and use hospital # k as the reference hospital. It is then possible to conduct an overall test to see if the effect of the hospital on outcome differs significantly among the hospitals. If so, one may proceed and examine the individual hospital coefficients.

When one is conducting a regression analysis or assessing the results of one conducted by others, it is important to be familiar with two concepts; unexplained variation and interaction.

5.3.2 Unexplained Variation

The purpose of using linear regression is to predict the value of a continuous outcome measure. To assess the usefulness of this prediction, one needs to relate the observed outcome to the predicted one, for instance by calculating the difference between the two. This difference is called a prediction error. Alternatively, the ratio between the predicted value and the observed outcome can be calculated. Analysis of the prediction error allows one to assess how much of the observed variation is actually explained by the regression equation. To illustrate how this may be achieved, we return to Example 5.1 (see also Table 5.1).

Example 5.5

In Example 5.1, we found the following linear regression function

$$\text{operating time} = 4.7 - 1.0 \cdot \text{sequence} \# \qquad (5.6)$$

We want to assess how well this regression function fits the observed values. We do that by comparing the observed variation relative to the regression line to the variation we would find if we were to disregard the linear trend. In the latter case, the linear model reduces to

$$\text{operation time} = a + 0.0 \text{sequence} \# = a \qquad (5.7)$$

This model states that all values are constant, except for random variation. Therefore, the error of an observation is its difference from the chosen constant, a. The value of a that minimises the sum of squares of the errors is the mean value of the observed values, $\bar{y} = 1.700$. Using this model, the squared error of, e.g., observation # 4 (see Table 5.1) is $(0.500 - 1.700)^2 = 1.440$. The sum of squares of these errors is referred to as the adjusted sum of squares ($TSS(adj)$) [13, p 78–9]. Table 5.1 shows $TSS(adj)$ and SSE. Because the former (14.300) is larger than the latter (4.300), we conclude that the linear function explains more of the variation of the data than a simple constant.

The ratio between SSE and $TSS(adj)$ may theoretically vary between 0, when there is no variation relative to the regression line, and 1 when the regression line is horizontal (see Equation (5.7)). In the first case, all of the variation has been explained by the regression equation, and in the last case, none of it has been. Therefore, $\frac{SSE}{TSS(adj)}$ may be viewed as that part of the adjusted total variation ($TSS(adj)$) that is not explained by the regression line. Consequently, $R^2 = (1 - \frac{SSE}{TSS(adj)})$ [13, p 79 and 82] is that part that *is* explained by the regression line. In multiple linear regression analysis, SSE is calculated using the same principle as in simple linear regression analysis. $TSS(adj)$ may be calculated as explained above. Therefore, $R^2 = (1 - \frac{SSE}{TSS(adj)})$ may be calculated in multiple regression analysis and used as a measure of the variation explained by the multiple linear regression equation.

5.3.3   Interaction

The other important concept is interaction. We define this concept and illustrate its meaning, using an invented example without random variation.

Assume that we observe two independent variables, X_1 and X_2, and one dependent one, Y. If the relationship between X_1 and Y depends on the value of X_2 and vice versa, we say that X_1 and X_2 interact. To examine if two continuous independent variables or one continuous variable and one categorical one interact, we define a new variable that is $X_3 = X_1 \cdot X_2$. If both variables are categorical, say binary, the interaction is calculated as a variable with four levels, corresponding to the four combinations $(0,0), (1,0), (0,1)$, and $(1,1)$. This new variable is a categorical variable with 4 levels. Therefore, it has to be changed into three binary variables. However, we will confine ourselves to an analysis of one continuous and one categorical independent variable. We have the following regression equation

$$Y_i = \alpha + \beta_1 X_{1i} + \beta_2 X_{2i} + \beta_3 X_{3i} + \varepsilon_i \qquad (5.8)$$

For simplicity we omit the index i in the following. Whether X_1 and X_2 interact or not may be tested. If β_3 does not deviate significantly from zero, it may be concluded that there is no interaction between X_1 and X_2.

Example 5.6

Figure 5.3 offers a graphical illustration of the concept of interaction. Frame (a) illustrates the situation where the binary variable X_1 and the

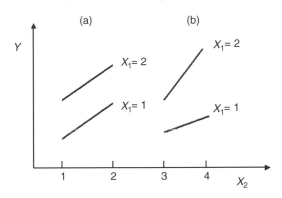

Y as a function of X_1 and X_2

Figure 5.3 Interaction between X_1 and X_2. Frame (a) illustrates lack of interaction (the two lines are parallel). Frame (b) shows example of interaction (the two lines are not parallel).

continuous variable X_2 do not interact. For both values of X_1 the slope of Y as a function of X_2 is the same, i.e., the lines are parallel; and for all values of X_2, the difference between the Y value obtained when $X_1 - 1$ and that obtained when $X_1 = 2$ is the same. Therefore, Y as a function of X_1 is independent of the value of X_2, and vice versa. Frame (b) illustrates a case of interaction between X_1 and X_2. The two lines are not parallel signifying that the slope depends on the value of X_1, and the distance between the two lines is not the same everywhere signifying that Y as a function of X_1 depends on the value of X_2.

5.3.4   Hierarchical Linear Regression

To explain the basic principles of hierarchical models, we will use a case story taken from the literature [14]. The aim of the study was to compare physicians, treating type II diabetic patients within a specified centre. The dependent variable was patient satisfaction. It may be argued that it should not be risk adjusted [15]. But that is a minor concern in this context. Each patient was asked to fill a questionnaire pertaining to his/her satisfaction with his/her physician. The answers of each patient were combined to obtain a satisfaction score, theoretically ranging from 0 to 100. The objective of the study was to assess if there is a difference across physicians in the mean outcome scores received, adjusted for the relationship between appropriate independent variables

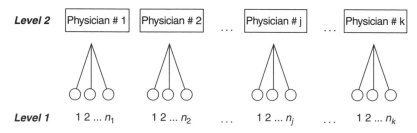

Figure 5.4 Illustrates the hierarchical structure of the problem presented in the study by Sullivan *et al.* [14]. Level 1 is the patient level, and level 2 is the physician level.

and the satisfaction score. To simplify matters, we will focus on a single patient-specific independent variable, namely the patient's age.

Figure 5.4 depicts the hierarchical nature of this study. At the highest level we have the physicians. They were sampled within the centre examined. Within each physician, patients (the primary level units) were sampled, their satisfaction scores measured, and their ages recorded. If the patient age is related to the patient satisfaction, we want to adjust for this relationship before we compare the mean satisfaction scores between physicians. The size of the patient samples varied considerably, ranging from 5 to 45 patients. Three types of models have been used for this kind of problem. We review all three models, in increasing order of refinement.

5.3.4.1 Single level model without provider effect

Until recently, this model has been the most commonly used in the scientific medical literature. It states that

$$Y_i = \alpha + \beta X_i + \varepsilon_i \tag{5.9}$$

where Y_i is the score measured in patient # i, i runs from 1 to n, and n is the total number of patients; α and β are the parameters of the linear relationship, X_i the patient's age, and ε_i a random deviation from the linear relationship between patient age and satisfaction score.

Using this model, one pools all patient values and uses them to estimate the relationship between patient age and satisfaction score. The predicted outcome of each individual patient is calculated using the resulting regression equation. Finally, the ratio between observed and predicted outcome (or the difference) is calculated for each physician, and the results compared between physicians. This approach has several shortcomings. In addition to the random variation, that is not incorporated in the model, there may be additional, unexplained variation that cannot be accounted for by the fixed parameters of the model. This includes variability between physicians and variability between patients, within physicians. In the above model this variation is pooled. Thus, a distinction is not made between patients and physicians.

5.3.4.2 The single level model with fixed provider effect

If one is only interested in the k physicians included in the study and not interested in making inferences about other physicians, one may use one of them as a reference and define $k - 1$ fixed parameters, representing the remaining $k - 1$ physicians. We, therefore, obtain the following model

$$Y_{ji} = \alpha + \beta X_{ji} + \sum_{v=1}^{k-1} \delta_v \mathrm{PH}_v + \varepsilon_{ji} \qquad (5.10)$$

where Y_{ji} is the score of the ith patient under physician # j, and X_{ji} is the patient's age; PH_v is 1 if $v = j$ and otherwise 0, and δ_v is the fixed effect of physician # v.

One shortcoming of a single level model is that all observations are assumed to be independent. However, studies often include clusters of observations that have a natural tendency to be similar within clusters.

5.3.4.3 Hierarchical (or multilevel or mixed) linear regression

A hierarchical model of the above problem may be developed as follows: We have k physicians. For each physician, e.g., the jth, we have $i = 1, \ldots, n_j$ patients. Y_{ji} is the dependent variable that corresponds to the ith patient for the jth physician. X_{ji} is the corresponding independent variable. We have the following model

$$Y_{ji} = \alpha_j + \beta_j X_{ji} + \varepsilon_{ji} \qquad (5.11)$$

where ε_{ji} is the random error. This model is referred to as a hierarchical regression model. Sometimes it is also called a multilevel regression model or a mixed model. It is often useful to centre the variable X_{ji} on its grand mean $\bar{X}_{..}$. Therefore, we express Equation (5.11) as

$$Y_{ji} = \alpha_j + \beta_j(X_{ji} - \bar{X}_{..}) + \varepsilon_{ji} \qquad (5.12)$$

In a hierarchical model one operates with a number of levels combined in a hierarchical structure. In the example there are two levels; the patient level and the physician level. Level 1 is the patient level. We will start with the physician level model (the level 2 model). There are k physicians. Each physician, e.g., the jth physician, is considered a unit sampled from a population of physicians that we want to investigate (in the example, the present and future physicians at the centre). The intercept α_j and the slope β_j in the level 2 model have general random structures in the paper by Sullivan et al. [14]. By this we mean that they may both be decomposed into a fixed component (fixed effect) that is common to all physicians and a random component that varies at random from one physician to the next one. Sullivan et al. found that the slope (β) had no random component, i.e., that it is the same for all physicians. The intercept, however, did have a significant general random structure. Therefore, we have

$$\alpha_j = g + \nu_j \tag{5.13}$$

where j goes from 1 to k and refers to the jth physician. Each physician's value consists of a fixed component (g, the grand mean of the population of physicians) and a random deviation (ν_j) from this mean. In statistics, ν_j is called a random effect. We assume that the random deviations follow a Gaussian distribution with mean 0 and variance ν^2. For a specified physician (physician # j), ν_j is an unknown constant, characterising this particular physician.

The level 1 model models the satisfaction score, characterising each patient. This score depends on the physician by whom the patient is being treated and the independent variables characterising the patient, in this case his/her age. Therefore, the level 1 model becomes

$$Y_{ji} = g + \nu_j + \beta(X_{ji} - \bar{X}_{..}) + \varepsilon_{ji} \tag{5.14}$$

Y_{ji} is the observed satisfaction score of the ith of those (n_j) patients belonging to physician number j; ν_j is the random effect due to the jth physician; β the fixed slope effect; X_{ji} the age of the ith patient under physician # j; and ε_{ji} is a random deviation from the expected value. It is distributed with mean 0 and variance σ^2.

Main distinctive features of hierarchical models The hierarchical model has three main distinctive features. It models differences between providers, it 'shrinks' the estimates of the providers' average outcomes, and it acknowledges the clustering of observations.

A Differences between providers   The hierarchical model explicitly recognises as many sources of variation in the data as there are levels in the model. For instance, if we have two levels- patient and hospital- the model includes two components of variation (1) within each hospital the variation of the patients' observed outcomes from the hospital's true average outcome and (2) the variation across hospitals in their true average outcomes.

At each level, the sources of variation may be random or systematic (fixed effect). At the patient level, systematic effects include risk factors such as age, co-morbidity, socioeconomic status, etc. At the hospital level, they may include volume (number of patients received per time unit), teaching status, etc.

B Shrinkage of estimates of provider outcomes   When there are three or more providers, the hierarchical model estimates their mean values using a compromise between two extremes: (1) they all have the same mean, namely the grand mean or (2) they each have a mean value calculated from the values within the group (the traditional unbiased estimate). The result is that the latter group means move towards the grand mean. This movement is the 'shrinkage' caused by the hierarchical model as compared to a non-hierarchical model. The smaller the sample size of a group is, the more its mean 'shrinks'.

C Clustering of observations   Studies often include clusters of observations that have a natural tendency to be similar within clusters. For instance, the patients treated by the same very skilled surgeon will all benefit from that surgeon's expertise. Similarly surgeons operating within the same hospital tend to produce similar results. They all operate under the same organisation and share the same facilities and resources. This natural similarity means that the outcomes of the units within a cluster are generally more correlated with each other than they are with the outcomes of units from other clusters. The hierarchical model explicitly acknowledges and provides estimates of these intra-class correlations. The larger the intra-class correlation is, the smaller is the effective sample size. This has a bearing on the confidence intervals of the provider effect that become wider.

For a review and discussion of various medical applications of multilevel modelling the reader is referred to [16–18]. The chapter 'Comparing outcomes across providers' by AS Ash, M Schwartz, and EA Pekoz, in the textbook by LI Iezzoni [1] provides an excellent and informal introduction to the topic.

Example 5.7

Table 5.4 shows a sample of the physicians examined in the study by Sullivan *et al.* [14]. The mean patient score of each physician is estimated as the unbiased group average (column 3) and again, using the hierarchical model, as the physician mean plus the random effect (column 4). The latter estimates are closer to the physician grand mean (68.0) than the unbiased group averages. In the example study by Sullivan *et al.* [14], the authors used the hierarchical model explained above (see Equations (5.13) and (5.14)).

We present their results in Table 5.5. This table shows the estimates of the parameters of the hierarchical model, the standard errors of the parameters, and the corresponding p-values. The variance of the population of physicians, v^2, is significantly different from 0. This means that the mean levels of the physicians differ significantly. Therefore, it makes sense to estimate the random effects. In Table 5.5 the estimated physician-specific random deviations from the grand mean (g) are shown for three of the 81 physicians included in the study. In each case, it has been tested if the random effect is significantly different from 0. The results of these tests are also shown. The fixed slope ($\hat{\beta}$), relating the deviation of a patient's age from the average, to

Table 5.4 Estimates of mean patient satisfaction scores of individual physicians, using individual sample means ($\bar{x}_j$) and a hierarchical model ($\hat{\alpha}_j$).

Physician # (j)	Sample size (n_j)	Individual sample means ($\bar{x}_j$)	Estimates based on hierarchical model ($\hat{\alpha}_j$)
5	28	71.4	70.5
1	21	69.6	68.9
Grand mean		68.0	68.0
6	45	67.9	67.8
8	11	66.6	67.2
7	16	65.1	66.8
81	23	56.8	62.1
3	25	54.0	60.3

Table 5.5 Estimates, standard errors, and p-values of the parameters of the model: $Y_{ji} = \alpha_j + \beta(X_{ji} - \bar{X}_{..}) + \varepsilon_{ji}$. For explanation of parameters, see text.

Parameter	Estimate	Standard error	p
$\hat{g}$	68.000	0.859	0.0001
v^2	24.780	8.387	0.0031
$\hat{\alpha}_1 - \hat{g}$	0.910	3.554	0.7970
$\hat{\alpha}_3 - \hat{g}$	−7.670	3.404	0.0245
$\hat{\alpha}_{81} - \hat{g}$	−5.870	3.476	0.0915
β	0.153	0.051	0.0027
$\hat{\sigma}^2$	524.930	19.650	0.0001

the satisfaction score, was significantly different from zero. The physician-specific level is $\hat{\alpha}_j$. It may be interpreted as the estimated score of a patient who is treated by this physician and has an age equal to the average.

One purpose of using a hierarchical model is to obtain the confidence interval of α_j, the individual physician level. Then, it may be determined if the interval includes some benchmark value, say the national average (see Chapter 7). If this is not the case, the physician is identified as an outlier, and the reason for this should be investigated. Implied in this approach is that k significance tests are performed, where k is the number of physicians. If the tests are independent and the significance level is p, the probability that at least one is erroneously classified as an outlier is not p, but 1 minus the probability that none of them are erroneously classified as an outlier, i.e., $1 - (1 - p)^k$. For example, if $p = 0.05$ and $k = 10$, the probability is $1 - (1 - 0.05)^{10} = 0.401$. This problem may be remedied by choosing a lower value of p. However, the approach may be problematic for two other reasons; (1) the assumption that the α_j follow a normal distribution is not particularly well founded, and (2) the outlying physicians that we want to identify may inflate the variance of the distribution and thereby hide all or some of the truly outlying physicians. The resolution of these problems is the topic of ongoing research [19].

In this section, we have dealt with continuous outcome measures. More often than not the outcome of interest is binary. This problem will be analysed in Section 5.4.

5.4 LOGISTIC REGRESSION ON BINARY DATA

The task in logistic regression is to estimate the probability of a binary outcome. This problem is approached by first translating it into a linear problem, solving it, and then, by using the reverse transformation, converting the result back to the original metric. We start with the single level model and proceed to explain the hierarchical model.

5.4.1 Single Level Logistic Regression Model

In the present context, this model is used to predict a patient's probability of experiencing the event studied, e.g., death following an operation or being assigned to a specified 'intervention' group. The variable of interest is the probability, $P(Y = 1) = p$, of the event. Various factors that influence this probability are the risk factors or independent variables. The probability p may be estimated as a proportion. If 30 patients out of 100 patients die, the probability (p) of death of future patients of this type may be estimated as $\frac{30}{100} = 0.3$. The multiple linear regression model is not applicable to describing the relationship between p and a number of independent variables. One of the reasons is that the possible values of p are confined to the interval $[0,1]$. To obtain a larger range of possible values, the odds are used in place of the probability. The odds are the probability (p) that a specified event takes place, divided by the probability $(1 - p)$ that it does not. The calculation of the odds, given the probability, and vice versa, may be done using the following equations

$$\text{odds} = \frac{p}{1 - p} \tag{5.15}$$

and

$$p = \frac{\text{odds}}{1 + \text{odds}} \tag{5.16}$$

By taking the logarithm of the odds, we obtain a variable that may attain values going from $-\infty$ to $+\infty$. Therefore, we use this transformation and relate $\log(\frac{p}{1-p})$ to the risk factors, using a linear regression technique. The risk factors may be continuous, categorical, or a mixture of both (see Section 5.1). For a specific patient, patient # i, we have $\log(\text{odds}_i) = \log(\frac{p_i}{1-p_i})$, also referred to as $\text{logit}(p_i)$. We have:

$$\text{logit}(p_i) = \alpha + \beta_1 X_{1i} + \beta_2 X_{2i} + \beta_3 X_{3i} + \cdots + \beta_p X_{pi} + \varepsilon_i \tag{5.17}$$

where p_i is the probability that patient # i experiences the event; α, $\beta_1, \ldots, \beta_p$ are the parameters of the regression equation, and X_{1i} through X_{pi} are the p independent variables or risk factors, observed in patient # i. ε_i is a random error. The latter quantity follows a binomial distribution. Therefore, special programmes are required to estimate the regression equation. We will analyse the data of Example 5.3 (see Table 5.2) using such a program and study the output.

Example 5.8

The analysis of the data set of Example 5.3 revealed that the application of PEEP was without influence on the odds of postoperative complication.

This is apparent from the results (see Table 5.6) of a logistic regression of the risk factors smoking status (pack-year), change in functional residual capacity (ΔFRC), duration of the operation (op-time), and the treatment variable PEEP on the logit of the probability of the occurrence of postoperative complication.

Table 5.6 depicts the estimated constant and the coefficients of pack-year, ΔFRC, op-time, and PEEP. The standard errors and the corresponding p-values are also shown. The coefficient of PEEP does not differ significantly from 0, at the 5% level of significance. The coefficients of the remaining independent variables all differ significantly from 0. Therefore, the application of PEEP is not significantly related to the occurrence of postoperative complications, given the values of the risk factors. However, the latter are significantly related to the occurrence of

Table 5.6 Output from regression of cigarette smoking in pack-year (pack-year$_i$), pre-operative functional residual capacity reduction (ΔFRC$_i$), operating time/minute (op-time$_i$), and peroperative application of end expiratory pressure (PEEP$_i$) on the logarithm of the odds of occurrence of postoperative complication (logit(p_i)).

Parameters[a]	Estimate	Standard error	p
α	−2.158	1.489	0.147
β_1	0.100	0.040	0.013
β_2	−2.312	0.931	0.013
β_3	0.011	0.005	0.023
β_4	0.121	0.915	0.895

[a] Parameters of the regression: $\text{logit}(p_i) = \alpha + \beta_1 \cdot \text{pack-year}_i + \beta_2 \cdot \Delta\text{FRC}_i + \beta_3 \, \text{op-time}_i + \beta_4 \, \text{PEEP}_i$.

complications. One may exclude PEEP from the model. Recalculating the regression equation without PEEP, we obtain the following equation

$$\widehat{\text{logit}}(p_i) = -2.065 + 0.099 \text{ pack-year}_i$$
$$- 2.317 \, \Delta\text{FRC}_i + 0.011 \text{ op-time}_i.$$

To calculate the odds corresponding to a given logit value, we calculate the exponential function of the logit since by definition $e^{\log(x)} = x$ and, therefore, $e^{\log\left(\frac{p}{1-p}\right)} = \frac{p}{1-p}$. Knowing the odds, one may calculate the corresponding probability. Assume, e.g., that we want to estimate the probability that patient # 1 (see Table 5.2) will develop postoperative complications. The smoking status of this patient is 10 pack-year, his/her ΔFRC is 2.69, and his/her op-time is 140 minutes. We have

$$\log(\widehat{\text{odds}}_1) = -2.065 + 0.099 \cdot 10 - 2.317 \cdot 2.69 + 0.011 \cdot 140 = -5.768.$$

His/her estimated odds of developing postoperative complications are $e^{-5.768} = 0.00313$. Using Equation (5.16), we estimate the probability p_1 as $\frac{0.00313}{1+0.00313} = 0.00312$.

To appreciate the implications of a logistic regression, it is useful to know how the coefficients ought to be interpreted. If the variable is continuous, $e^{\text{coefficient}}$ is the ratio between the odds (OR) of two patients. The first patient has a value that is one unit higher than that of the second one. It is assumed that the values of the other independent variables are the same in both patients. For instance, for fixed values of the other variables, the OR of two patients differing in smoking status by one pack-year is $e^{0.099} = 1.104$. If they differ by 10 pack-years, the OR is $e^{0.099 \cdot 10} = 2.691$, etc. It is assumed that the relationship between the continuous variable and logit(p_i) is linear.

When the dependent variable is categorical, $e^{\text{coefficient}}$ is the ratio between the odds of a patient, belonging to the category, and those of a patient, belonging to the reference category, provided that the values of the other independent variables are fixed. A binary variable is coded as 1 or 0 (as is an indicator variable resulting from the splitting of a categorical variable into binary variables, see Section 5.1). Therefore, the impact of a binary risk factor may be compared to that of another one, by comparing the corresponding two coefficients. If the risk factor is a continuous variable, the value of the coefficient depends on the unit chosen (e.g., going from a unit of one mole per litre, to one of 100 moles per litre, the coefficient changes by a factor of 100). Clearly, the coefficients of different continuous risk factors, representing different types of quantities, cannot be meaningfully compared.

Sometimes, the OR corresponding to a coefficient and the 95 % confidence interval of the OR are presented in computer outputs. Since $e^0 = 1$, it may be concluded (as a rule of thumb) that the coefficient differs significantly from zero if 1 is not contained in the 95 % confidence interval of the OR.

5.4.2 Unexplained Variation

When the outcome measure is continuous, the explained variation may be assessed as R^2, as explained in Example 5.5. Since R^2 of the logistic model is always substantially less than 1, even with a perfect model, R^2 is not appropriate to use. However, appropriate measures of explained variation for binary dependent variables do exist [20] although they are seldom calculated or reported. For example, a more useful measure is

$$R_G^2 = \frac{\sum_{i=1}^{n} \hat{p}_i^2 - n\bar{p}^2}{n\bar{p}(1 - \bar{p})} \tag{5.18}$$

where $\hat{p}_i$ is the estimated probability from the logistic regression [20] that patient number i experiences the event of interest, and $\bar{p} = \frac{\sum_{i=1}^{n} y_i}{n}$ where y_i is the value of Y_i, the binary outcome measure of patient # i.

Example 5.9

This example is constructed using data from the study of surgical patients, described in Example 5.8. Table 5.2 shows for each of the 40 patients the estimated probability of experiencing postoperative complication as calculated using the regression equation (see table 5.6)

$$\widehat{\text{logit}}(p_i) = -2.158 + 0.100 \text{ pack-year}_i - 2.312 \text{ } \Delta\text{FRC}_i$$
$$+ 0.011 \text{ op-time}_i + 0.121 \text{ PEEP}_i.$$

The table also shows the square of each of these probabilities and the corresponding sum of squared probabilities. Since 16 of the 40 patients developed postoperative complications, $\bar{p} = \frac{16}{40} = 0.4$. From Table 5.2, we have that $\sum_{i=1}^{40} \hat{p}_i^2 = 10.828$ and $n = 40$. When we insert these values in Equation (5.18), we obtain

$$R_G^2 = \frac{10.828 - 40 \cdot 0.4^2}{40 \cdot 0.4 \cdot (1 - 0.4)} = 0.461.$$

In this case, $100 - 46.1 = 53.9$ % of the total variation is not explained.

5.4.3 Interaction

Interaction in logistic regression is defined and dealt with in the same way as in regression on a continuous outcome measure.

5.4.4 Hierarchical Logistic Regression Model

Before we proceed to explain the hierarchical logistic regression model, we first review the single level logistic regression models. Then, we present an example where the hierarchical model has been applied. For a review of the various types of models see the paper by DeLong *et al.* [21].

5.4.4.1 Single level model without provider representation

Until recently, a single level model without provider representation was often used in the literature. Under this approach, a logistic regression equation is first developed from all the patient data. Using this equation, the probability of an adverse event is estimated in each patient. The sum of these probabilities, calculated for each provider, estimates the expected number of patients experiencing the adverse event (E_j, where j is the provider number). O_j is the corresponding observed number. $\frac{O_j}{E_j}$ is compared between the providers.

5.4.4.2 Single level model including fixed provider effect

This model includes the provider effect as a fixed effect. We have the following model

$$\text{logit}(p_{ji}) = \alpha + \sum_{b=1}^{k-1} \delta_b \text{PH}_b + \sum_{v=1}^{m} \beta_v (X_{vji} - \bar{X}_{v..}) + \varepsilon_{ji} \qquad (5.19)$$

where p_{ji} is the probability that patient # i, treated by provider # j $(j = 1, \ldots, k)$, where k is the total number of providers, experiences an adverse event; X_{vji} is the vth risk factor out of a total of m risk factors observed in patient # i, treated by provider # j; PH_h is 1 for $h = j$ and otherwise 0. $\bar{X}_{v..}$ is the mean of risk factor # v, and ε_{ji} is a random deviation. According to this model, the providers have different intercepts. It is assumed that all observations are independent, and inferences are made only about the providers actually studied.

5.4.4.3 Hierarchical models

It is also possible to use hierarchical logistic models. Their technical implementation is different from that of models for continuous outcome measures. However, conceptually they do not differ from the latter models. We will present the results of a study of the 30-day mortality of patients suffering from AMI.

Example 5.10

The study included 19 585 patients with AMI admitted to 163 hospitals in Ontario [22]. The hospitals were classified into 4 peer groups: teaching hospitals and three categories of non-teaching hospitals. The latter were subdivided according to volume (patients treated per year) into 3 groups receiving 1 to 50, 51 to 250, and more than 250 patients per year, respectively. Adjustment for differences in case mix was done, using a number of risk factors including age, sex, and various measures of cardiac complications and co-morbid status (see legend to Table 5.7).
  The model used was

$$\text{logit}(p_{ji}) = \beta_{oj} + \sum_{v=1}^{m} \beta_v (X_{vji} - \bar{X}_{v..}) + \varepsilon_{ji} \qquad (5.20)$$

where p_{ji} is the probability of 30-day mortality for patient # i, treated in hospital # j; and X_{vji} denotes risk factor # v measured in this patient $(v = 1$ to $m)$.
  $\bar{X}_{v..}$ is the mean of risk factor # v and ε_{ji} is a random deviation. β_{oj} is the effect of the hospital for a patient presenting with average risk factor combinations. The level 2 model is

$$\beta_{oj} = \alpha_o + \alpha_1 \delta_1 + \alpha_2 \delta_2 + \alpha_3 \delta_3 + \tau_j \qquad (5.21)$$

Where α_o is the mean value of teaching hospitals. δ_1 is 1 if the hospital is a non-teaching large volume hospital, and otherwise 0, δ_2 is 1 if the

Table 5.7 The estimates of the coefficients of hospital characteristics[a] from a hierarchical regression analysis[b] of healthcare provider (hospital) (random effect), hospital characteristics (fixed effect), and patient characteristics[c] on $\text{logit}(p)$[d] [22].

Parameter	Estimate	p
α_o (mean intercept)	−3.030	0.001
v^2 (variance of random intercept)	0.044	0.001
α_1 (large volume)	0.300	0.004
α_2 (medium volume)	0.460	0.001
α_3 (small volume)	0.570	0.001

[a] The hospitals were classified into four peer groups: Teaching hospitals (reference category) and three categories of non-teaching hospitals, large volume (more than 250 patients treated per year), medium volume (51 to 250 patients treated per year), and small volume hospitals (1 to 50 patients treated per year).
[b] The hierarchical model included two levels, patients (level 1) and hospitals (level 2).
[c] Age, sex, congestive heart failure, cardiogenic shock, arrhythmia, pulmonary oedema, diabetes with complications, stroke, renal disease, and malignancy.
[d] p-value.

hospital is a non-teaching medium volume hospital, and otherwise 0, and δ_3 is 1 if the hospital is a non-teaching small volume hospital, and otherwise 0. The reference, against which the hospitals are compared, is a teaching hospital. τ_j is the hospital-specific random effect that is assumed to follow a normal distribution, with mean 0 and variance v^2. τ_j is the logarithm of the odds ratio of mortality at the given hospital compared to an average-mortality hospital that shares the same hospital characteristics. For instance for a large volumes hospital we have the odds ratio $\frac{e^{\alpha_1 + \tau_j}}{e^{\alpha_1}} = e^{\tau_j}$. $\log(e^{\tau_j}) = \tau_j$.

Table 5.7 shows the estimates of the above level 2 parameters and the corresponding p-values. The random effects as well as all the fixed peer group effects are highly significant. For a patient with average risk factor values who is treated at an average teaching hospital, we have $\widehat{\text{logit}}(p) = -3.030$. The estimated odds are $e^{-3.030} = 0.0483$, and the estimated probability of dying is $\frac{0.0483}{1+0.0483} = 0.0461$. By contrast, for a similar patient treated at an average small volume hospital, the estimated odds are $e^{(-3.03+0.57)} = 0.0854$ (see Table 5.7), and $\hat{p}$ is 0.0787. If the patient is treated at a teaching hospital characterised by $\hat{\tau}_j$ being 0.5, the estimated odds are $e^{(-3.03+0.5)} = 0.0797$ and $\hat{p} = 0.0738$.

Figure 5.5 from [22] shows the distributions of hospital-specific log odds of death, stratified by peer group. The overlap between these distributions is considerable. The conclusion from this study, given the assumptions, is that peer group is a significant factor. However, for a given peer group, the hospitals differ significantly. Adjusting for peer

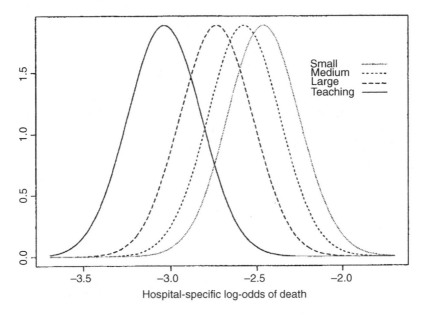

Figure 5.5 Reproduced from Austin PC, Alter DA, Anderson GM, Tu JV with permission. Impact of choice of benchmark on the conclusions of hospital report cards. Am Heart J 2004; 148:1041–46.

group, the authors found one low outlying hospital. When they did not adjust, they found 3 high outliers and 4 low ones.

5.5 ASSESSING THE QUALITY OF A REGRESSION MODEL

Once a regression model is developed, it is necessary to assess its quality. The principles applied for the multiple regression model and the logistic regression model are similar. Since the latter is by far the most popular model in medical literature, we will use this model to illustrate the principles. We want to emphasise that it is not our intention with this section to teach the reader how to develop and quality control a model. However, to critically assess the literature, it is necessary to know what to look for.

The quality may be related to events per predictor variable, conformity with linear gradient, test for interactions, collinearity, goodness-of-fit measures, validation, statistical significance, and proper documentation [23].

5.5.1   Events per Predictor Variable

If there are too few events per independent predictor variable included in a model, the results may become unreliable. A useful rule of thumb comes from simulation experiments [24]. It suggests that the number of the less frequent of the two events divided by the number of predictor variables included in the model should be at least 10. For instance, if a study includes 200 patients, and 20 of the patients died, it must not include more than $\frac{20}{10} = 2$ predictor variables.

5.5.2   Conformity with Linear Gradients for Continuous Variables

Any given change in a continuous (or multinomial ranked) predictor variable ought to have an effect on the logit that is of the same magnitude, regardless of the value of the predictor variable. This must be checked because it is assumed in the model. One may add that converting a continuous variable into a binary one is not recommended because it represents a loss of information and there is the danger that the model becomes incorrectly specified [25].

5.5.3   Tests for Interactions

In general, when the sample size is modest, the decision to consider interactions should be governed by prior knowledge of the domain. In any event, the significance of the interaction should be measured and reported.

5.5.4   Collinearity

If two predictor variables are highly correlated with each other, it presents problems for a regression analysis [26]. Therefore, explicit tests for collinearity ought to be undertaken.

5.5.5   Goodness-of-Fit Measures

These include calibration, discrimination, and various regression statistics. The latter are used to reveal the effect of individual subjects on the estimated model [10]. In the following, we will expand on the former two measures.

5.5.5.1   Calibration

Calibration may be defined as the ability to assign appropriate risks among patients whose experience the model simulates [27]. A model is calibrated if the distribution of the estimated risks does not differ significantly from that of the observed outcomes. Comparing the predicted and observed outcomes assesses the calibration. The predicted outcome for a given group of patients is calculated by using the model to calculate the probability of experiencing the outcome in each of the patients and adding these probabilities.

Example 5.11

Table 5.2 column 9 from Example 5.3 shows the predicted probability of experiencing postoperative complications as calculated using the regression of ΔFRC_i, op-time$_i$, and pack-year$_i$ and $PEEP_i$ on logit(p_i). The data have been sorted in ascending order, according to the probability. To illustrate the principle, we have grouped the data into 10 subgroups, each comprising four consecutive patients (see Table 5.8).

The expected number of patients with complication in the first group (see Table 5.2) is $0.003 + 0.003 + 0.006 + 0.028 = 0.040$. Therefore, the expected number without complication is $4.000 - 0.040 = 3.960$. The corresponding observed values are 0 and 4 (see Table 5.8). The results of these calculations for all 10 subgroups are shown in Table 5.8.

Table 5.8 Predicted versus observed number of patients with postoperative complication.

Group	Observed number with complication	Predicted number with complication	Observed number without complication	Predicted number without complication
1	0	0.040	4	3.960
2	0	0.180	4	3.820
3	0	0.281	4	3.719
4	2	0.575	2	3.425
5	2	1.087	2	2.913
6	0	1.707	4	2.293
7	1	2.084	3	1.916
8	3	2.777	1	1.223
9	4	3.365	0	0.635
10	4	3.903	0	0.097

It may be tested if the distribution of the observed numbers differs significantly from that of the expected numbers. This is the Hosmer Lemeshow test [10]. If the p-value of this test is reasonably large, it is taken as evidence of acceptable calibration. In the actual case $p = 0.214$.

In the example, the (nonsignificant) trend is that the predicted number of patients with complication is too high in the lower range and too low in the upper range (see Table 5.8). This is not an unusual pattern, and, if it is significant and pronounced, it may have unfortunate consequences. For example, if one were to compare the observed number of deaths following an operation to the predicted number of deaths and use a model where the above pattern is significant, the predicted number of deaths in high-risk patients would be underestimated, while the pre- dicted number would be overestimated in low-risk patients. Therefore, using this model one would treat healthcare providers with high-risk patients unfairly because their mortality would exceed the predicted one. This, in turn, may encourage rejection of high-risk patients. Conse- quently, a model with this kind of lack of calibration is not acceptable.

A model initially well calibrated (and verified, see later) may be applied to materials other than those used to develop the model, either from another institution or from the same institution, at a much later date. If there is now a significant discrepancy between predicted and observed outcomes, showing poor calibration, several approaches are possible. One may calibrate the model in various ways, or, alternatively, use one's own patient data to develop a new model, either based on the same quantities as the original model or on a new combination of quantities [21]. However, in doing so one loses the historic perspective.

5.5.5.2 Discrimination

The fact that a model is well calibrated does not necessarily imply that the estimated probability is useful as a discriminating quantity. A dis- criminating quantity D, may be used to classify patients into two groups: those who are predicted to experience some event of interest (group # 1) and those who are not (group # 2). The estimated probability of experi- encing the event ($\hat{p}$) is a discriminator. Prior to the classification a discriminating value (d) must be chosen. Patients who have estimated probabilities $> d$ are classified into group # 1, and the rest into group # 2. Usually $d = 0.5$ is chosen. To assess the usefulness of a classification rule, we calculate its sensitivity and specificity. Assume the outcome is death following an operation. The sensitivity is defined as the number of patients who were correctly predicted to die over the total number who died. The specificity is defined as number of patients who were correctly classified as survivors over the total number of survivors. Depending on the expected consequences of misclassifications, values of d other than 0.5 may be chosen.

A complete discrimination may be obtained if the group of survivors is completely separated from the group of dead, in terms of their values of D (see Figure 5.6 frame (a)). If the ratio between surviving and dead patients is the same for all values of D (see Figure 5.6, frame (b)), D is useless as a discriminator.

In general, if the chosen discriminating value (d-low) is sufficiently small, all patients will be classified as dead, and if it is sufficiently large (d-$high$), all will be classified as survivors (see Figure 5.6). One may vary the value of D from d-low to d-$high$, calculate the sensitivity and specificity (or 1 − specificity) for each value, and plot the results in a coordinate system, with sensitivity as the y-axis and 1 − specificity as the x-axis. The resulting curve is the receiver operating characteristic (ROC) curve [28, 29]. If the discrimination is optimal (case (a) in Figure 5.6), the area under this curve (the ROC-area) is 1. If there is no discrimination

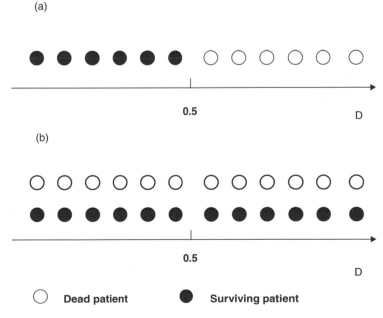

Figure 5.6 Complete discrimination (frame (a)) by the discriminator D (the predicted probability that a patient dies) between patients who die and those who do not versus no discrimination at all (frame (b)).

(case (b) in Figure 5.6) the area is 0.5. Therefore, one may grade a discriminator by calculating its ROC-area and judge its value on a scale from 0.5 to 1.

5.5.6   Validity

Validity may be defined as "the demonstration that the predictive accuracy of the model is similar when it is applied to a different group of patients than those used in the construction of the model" [27]. To assess the validity of a model, the following procedure is often followed: one half of the patients are randomly assigned to a learning set and the rest to a test set. The model is developed using the learning set and then applied on the test set. This method is called cross validation. If the calibration and discrimination of the test set are little degraded as compared to those of the learning set, the model has been validated. This approach requires a substantial number of cases. Other approaches are also possible [30].

5.5.7   Statistical Significance

The statistical significance of the null hypothesis that a coefficient is 0 may be tested for each coefficient in the model. It may also be tested if the complete model is significantly better than a reduced model with some of the coefficients set equal to 0. There are various types of tests, and the specific test applied should be reported [23].

5.5.8   Documentation

It is important that it is documented how variables have been selected for inclusion in the model. Were they selected based on earlier research or based on the observed association with the outcome measure? Since the coefficient of a predictor variable depends on how it was coded, appropriate description of the coding ought to be supplied. Finally, the procedure used to determine which variables were included in the model ought to be explicitly stated, preferably with some motivation for the appropriateness of the choice [23].

Techniques other than those described above are available, e.g., artificial intelligence (AI) [31]. AI has a number of theoretical advantages as compared to logistic regression. However, it requires large databases and does not have convenient features like odds ratio and confidence intervals. An analysis of 80 000 coronary artery bypass patients using AI failed to improve upon the ROC curve of logistic regression in risk prediction [32].

In the following two chapters, we illustrate how the above tools may be applied to risk-adjust the results of a single healthcare provider over time (Chapter 6) and the results of several providers who are being compared simultaneously (Chapter 7).

REFERENCES

[1] Iezzoni LI (ed). Risk Adjustment for Measuring Healthcare Outcomes. Health Administration Press, Chicago, 1997.

[2] Clark TG, Bradburn MJ, Love SB, and Altman DG. Survival analysis part I: basic concepts and first analysis. Br J Cancer 2003; 89:232–8.

[3] Bradburn MJ, Clark TG, Love SB, and Altman DG. Survival analysis part II: multivariate data analysis – an introduction to concepts and methods. Br J Cancer 2003; 89:431–6.

[4] Bradburn MJ, Clark TG, Love SB, and Altman DG. Survival analysis part III: multivariate data analysis – choosing a model and assessing its adequacy and fit. Br J Cancer 2003; 89:605–11.

[5] Clark TG, Bradburn MJ, Love SB, and Altman DG. Survival analysis part IV: further concepts and methods in survival analysis. Br J Cancer 2003; 89:781–6.

[6] Harrell FE, Jr. Regression Modeling Strategies with Applications to Linear Models, Logistic Regression, and Survival Analysis. Springer-Verlag, New York, 2001.

[7] Wetterslev J, Hansen EG, Roikjaer O, Kanstrup IL, and Heslet L. Optimizing perioperative compliance with PEEP during upper abdominal surgery: effects on perioperative oxygenation and complications in patients without preoperative cardiopulmonary dysfunction. Eur J Anaesthesiol 2001; 18:358–65.

[8] Grunkemeier GI, Zerr KJ, and Jin R. Cardiac surgery report cards making the grade. Ann Thorac Surg 2001; 72:1845–8.

[9] Harrell FE, Lee KL, and Mark DB. Multivariable prognostic models issues in developing models, evaluating assumptions and adequacy, and measuring and reducing errors. Stat Med 1996; 15:361–87.

[10] Hosmer DL, and Lemeshow S. Applied Logistic Regression. John Wiley and Sons Inc, New York, 2000.

[11] Steyerberg EW, Eijkemans MJ, Harrell FE, Jr., and Habbema JD. Prognostic modelling with logistic regression analysis: a comparison of selection and estimation methods in small data sets. Stat Med 2000; 19:1059–79.

[12] Spiegelhalter JD. Probabilistic prediction in patient management and clinical trials. Stat Med 1986; 5:421–33.

[13] Gunst RF, and Mason RL. Regression Analysis and its Application. Marcel Decker, New York, 1980.

[14] Sullivan LM, Dukes KA, and Losina E. Tutorial in biostatistics and introduction to hierarchical linear modelling. Stat Med 1999; 18:855–88.

[15] Press I. The measure of quality. Q Manage Health Care 2004; 13:202–9.

[16] Christiansen CL, and Morris CN. Improving the statistical approach to health care provider profiling. Ann Intern Med 1997; 127:764–8.

[17] Goldstein H, Browne W, and Rasbash J: Tutorial in biostatistics multilevel modelling of medical data. Stat Med 2002; 21:3291–3315.

[18] Greenland S. Principles of multilevel modelling. Int J Epidemiol 2000; 29:158–67.

[19] Ohlssen DI, Sharples LD, and Spiegelhalter DJ. Flexible random-effects models using Bayesian semi-parametric models: applications to institutional comparisons. Stat Med 2006; (in press).

[20] Mittlbock M, and Schemper M. Explained variation for logistic regression. Stat Med 1996; 15:1987–97.

[21] DeLong ER, Peterson ED, DeLong DM, Muhlbaier LH, Hackett S, and Mark DB. Comparing risk-adjustment methods for provider profiling. Stat Med 1997; 16:2645–64.

[22] Austin PC, Alter DA, Anderson GM, and Tu JV. Impact of choice of benchmark on the conclusions of hospital report cards. Am Heart J 2004; 148:1041–6.

[23] Bagley SC, White H, and Golomb BA. Logistic regression in the medical literature: standards for use and reporting, with particular attention to one medical domain. J Clin Epidemiol 2001; 54:979–85.

[24] Peduzzi P, Concalo J, Kemper E, Holford TR, and Feinstein AR. A simulation study of the number of events per variable in logistic regression analysis. J Clin Epidemiol 1996; 49:1373–9.

[25] Deeks JJ, Dinnes J, D'Amico R, Sowden AJ, Sakarovitch C, Song F, Petticrew M, and Altman DG. Evaluating non-randomised intervention studies. Health Technol Assess 2003; 7:1-173.

[26] Feinstein AE. Multivariable Analysis: an Introduction. Yale University Press, New Haven, 1996.

[27] Anderson RP, Jin R, and Grunkemeier GL. Understanding logistic regression analysis in clinical reports: an introduction. Ann Thorac Surg 2003; 75:753–7.

[28] Grunkemeier Gl, and Jin R. Receiver operating characteristic curve analysis of clinical risk models. Ann Thorac Surg 2001; 72:323–6.

[29] Hanley JA, and McNeil BJ. The meaning and use of the area under a receiver operating characteristic (ROC) curve. Radiology 1982; 143:29–36.

[30] Efron B, and Tibshirani RJ. An Introduction to the Bootstrap. Chapman and Hall, New York, 1993.

[31] Baxt WG. Application of artificial neural networks to clinical medicine. Lancet 1995; 346:1135–8.

[32] Lippmann RP, and Shahian DM. Coronary artery bypass risk prediction using neural networks. Ann Thorac Surg 1997; 63:1635–43.

6

Risk-Adjusted Control Charts

In Chapter 5 we reviewed various techniques that may be used to adjust for case-mix differences. We apply these techniques when constructing risk-adjusted control charts. These charts may be used when outcome measures, e.g., death and morbidity, are monitored over time. With few exceptions [1, 2, 3] the research within this area has focused on the occurrence of an adverse event (mainly death following some surgical procedure), and consequently the outcome measure is either binary (e.g., patient dead or alive) or a count (e.g., the number of patients who died during a specified period). Therefore, we will focus on binary and count outcome measures in this chapter. For ease of terminology and without any loss of generality, we will use the term 'death' instead of 'occurrence of an adverse event'. We first discuss various types of risk adjustment and then present several risk-adjusted control charts.

6.1 RISK ADJUSTMENT

The most common approach to risk adjustment is to estimate the probability of death of each individual patient using a score (e.g., the Parsonnet score [4] for surgical patients) or the result obtained using a logistic regression model relating probability of death to patient factors.

Table 6.1 shows the values of the Parsonnet risk score (V_{ij}) measured in 11 patients prior to cardiac surgery (the data are invented, but consistent with data from the literature [5]). A risk model derived from a logistic regression analysis of a number of potential risk factors including

Statistical Development of Quality in Medicine   P. Winkel and N. F. Zhang
© 2007 John Wiley & Sons, Ltd

Table 6.1 Predicted probability of death within 30 days following cardiac surgery and various derived quantities in each of 11 patients. Prediction was calculated using a logistic regression equation.[a]

Sample # (i)	Patient # (i)	Parsonnet score	$\widehat{\text{logit}(p_{ij})}$[b]	$\widehat{\text{odds}}_{ij}$[c]	$\hat{p}_{ij}$[d]	$(1 - \hat{p}_{ij})$	$\hat{p}_{ij}(1 - \hat{p}_{ij})$	Y_{ij}[e]	$Y_{ij} - \hat{p}_{ij}$	$\Sigma(Y_{ij} - \hat{p}_{ij})$
1	1	7.0	-3.131	0.0437	0.0418	0.9582	0.0401	1	0.9582	0.9582
1	2	8.0	-3.054	0.0472	0.0450	0.9550	0.0430	1	0.9550	1.9132
1	3	13.3	-2.646	0.0709	0.0662	0.9338	0.0618	0	-0.0662	1.8470
1	4	12.0	-2.746	0.0642	0.0603	0.9397	0.0567	0	-0.0603	1.7867
1	5	16.0	-2.438	0.0873	0.0803	0.9197	0.0739	0	-0.0803	1.7064
2	1	20.0	-2.130	0.1188	0.1062	0.8938	0.0949	0	-0.1062	1.6002
2	2	34.0	-1.052	0.3492	0.2588	0.7412	0.1918	0	-0.2588	1.3414
2	3	41.0	-0.513	0.5987	0.3745	0.6255	0.2342	1	0.6255	1.9669
2	4	71.0	1.797	6.0315	0.8578	0.1422	0.1220	1	0.1422	2.1091
2	5	27.0	-1.591	0.2037	0.1692	0.8308	0.1406	0	-0.1692	1.9399
2	6	18.0	-2.284	0.1019	0.0925	0.9075	0.0839	0	-0.0925	1.8474

[a] $\widehat{\text{logit}(p_{ij})} = -3.67 + 0.077V_{ij}$, where $\hat{p}_{ij}$ is the estimated probability, V_{ij} the Parsonnet score, j the patient group number, and i the patient number.

[b] $\widehat{\text{logit}(p_{ij})} = \log(\widehat{\text{odds}}_{ij})$.

[c] $\widehat{\text{odds}}_{ij} = \frac{\hat{p}_{ij}}{1 - \hat{p}_{ij}}$.

[d] $\hat{p}_{ij}$ is the estimated probability that patient # i in sample # j dies.

[e] Y_{ij} is 1 if patient # i from sample # j dies and 0 otherwise.

the score and based on data from a centre for cardiac surgery [5] relates the 30-day mortality to the Parsonnet score as follows

$$\widehat{\text{logit}}(p_{ij}) = -3.67 + 0.077V_{ij} \qquad (6.1)$$

where ij refers to the ith patient in the jth patient sample. Using this model, logit (p_{ij}), the odds, and risk of death (p_{ij}) during the first 30 days following cardiac surgery have been estimated for each patient and shown in Table 6.1. For example, for patient # 1 in sample # 1, we have $\widehat{\text{logit}}(p_{11}) = -3.67 + 0.077 \cdot 7 = -3.131$. The corresponding odds are $e^{-3.131} = 0.0437$. Using Equation (5.16) we may calculate $\hat{p}_{11}$ as $\frac{0.0437}{1+0.0437} = 0.0418$. It is now hypothesised that $P(Y_{11} = 1)$, the probability that the patient dies, follows a discrete probability distribution with a parameter $p = \hat{p}_{11}$. If the patient actually died, the observed result would be 1, and the difference between the observed and 'expected' result would be $1 - 0.0418 = 0.9582$, and if he/she survived, it would be $0 - 0.0418 = -0.0418$. If several patients are observed, the number expected to die is calculated as the sum of these estimated probabilities. This measure may be related to the observed number of deaths.

An alternative approach to risk adjustment is to calculate the mortality rate in a reference group of patients who belong to the same category as the patient in question. For instance, Grigg and Farewell [6] divided the patients seen per year by a single general practitioner (GP) into 10 groups according to age and sex. They used the annual mortality rate for all of England and Wales (the death rate of all patients seen by GPs during the year) in each of these categories to adjust for age- and sex-dependent risk differences between the groups. Assume (as an invented example) that the mortality rate for females between 65 and 75 during a given year was 0.04, and during this year the GP saw 150 patients of this type. The expected number of death per year within the category would be $0.04 \cdot 150 = 6$ death/year. In this case, it is hypothesised that the number of deaths per year for this type of patients follows a Poisson distribution with parameter $\lambda_0 = 6$ death/year. If, e.g., 8 patients of this category actually died, the observed minus expected number of deaths would be $8 - 6 = 2$ death/year.

6.2   RISK-ADJUSTED CONTROL CHARTS

We review one risk-adjusted Shewhart chart (the p chart), four risk-adjusted time-weighted control charts (the variable life-adjusted display

Table 6.2 The risk-adjusted sample statistic and control limits (when applicable) of the p chart, the variable life adjusted display (VLAD), the sequential probability ratio test (SPRT) chart, and the cumulative sum (CUSUM) chart.

Type of control chart	Sample statistic	Control limits
p chart[a]	$\frac{O_j}{n_j}$ $(n_j > 1)$	$\frac{1}{n_j}\left[E_j \pm k\sqrt{\sum_{i=1}^{n_j}\hat{p}_{ij}(1-\hat{p}_{ij})}\right]$
VLAD	$S_j = S_{j-1} + [O_j - E_j]$	n.a.
SPRT chart	$S_j^b = S_{j-1} + W_j^c$	$\text{UCL}^d = \log(\frac{1-\beta^e}{\alpha^f})$
		$\text{LCL} = \log(\frac{\beta}{1-\alpha})$
CUSUM chart	$S_j = \max\{0; S_{j-1} + W_j\}$ or $S_j = \min\{0; S_{j-1} + W_j\}$ or both	Define in-control ARL and out-of-control ARL and find the control limit(s)

[a] O_j is the number of deaths in sample # j, E_j the expected number of deaths in sample # j, n_j the number of patients in sample # j, and $\hat{p}_{ij}$ the estimated probability that patient # i in sample # j dies.
[b] usually $S_0 = 0$.
[c] $W_j = Y_j\log(OR) - \log(1-\hat{p}_{j0}+OR\hat{p}_{j0})$ where $OR = \frac{\hat{p}_{j1}(1-\hat{p}_{j0})}{\hat{p}_{j0}(1-\hat{p}_{j1})}$, $\hat{p}_{j0}$ is the estimated probability that patient # j dies under the null hypothesis H_0, and $\hat{p}_{j1}$ the estimated probability that patient # j dies under the alternative hypothesis H_1.
[d] UCL = upper control limit.
[e] β = the error rate with which H_0 is accepted in favour of H_1.
[f] α = the error rate with which H_1 is accepted in favour of H_0.
[g] LCL = lower control limit.

(VLAD), the sequential probability ratio test (SPRT) chart, the resetting SPRT chart (RSPRT), and the cumulative sum (CUSUM) chart). Table 6.2 presents an overview of four of these charts.

6.2.1 Risk-Adjusted p Chart

This chart has no centreline since the expected death rate varies from sample to sample, and each sample has its own control limits [7]. The idea behind this chart is that the sum of estimated probabilities of death calculated for individuals belonging to a given sample of patients is used to estimate the expected number of deaths (E_j) among these patients. We define the random variable X_{ij} to be 1 for death with probability p_{ij} and 0 for survival with probability $(1-p_{ij})$ for the ith patient in the jth sample. We define $Y_j = \frac{\sum_{i=1}^{n_j}X_{ij}}{n_j}$ where n_j is the number of patients in sample # j. $E_j = \sum_{i=1}^{n_j}p_{ij}$. Estimators of the expected value and the standard deviation of Y_j are $\frac{E_j}{n_j} = \frac{\sum_{i=1}^{n_j}\hat{p}_{ij}}{n_j}$ and $\frac{\sqrt{\sum_{i=1}^{n_j}\hat{p}_{ij}(1-\hat{p}_{ij})}}{n_j}$, respectively (see Table 6.2). The control limits for each sample may be calculated as shown in Table 6.2.

Example 6.1

We will analyse the two patient samples presented in Table 6.1. First, we calculate a conventional p chart without risk adjustment. The overall death rate is $\frac{4}{11} = 0.3636$ since 4 out of 11 patients died ($\Sigma\Sigma y_{ij} = 4$). The death rates in the two samples are $\frac{2}{5} = 0.4$ and $\frac{2}{6} = 0.33$, respectively, and the corresponding standard deviations are $\sqrt{\frac{0.3636(1-0.3636)}{5}} = 0.2151$ and $\sqrt{\frac{0.3636(1-0.3636)}{6}} = 0.1964$ (see Equations (2.36) and (2.37)). It is obvious that if we were to use the usual p chart for variable sample size, neither death rate would be outside its control limits.

For comparison we calculate the risk-adjusted expected death rate and corresponding control limits of each of the two patient samples. For sample # 1 we have $\frac{E_1}{n_1} = \frac{\Sigma \hat{p}_{i1}}{n_1} = \frac{0.0418+0.0450+0.0662+0.0603+0.0803}{5} = 0.0587$. The corresponding result for sample # 2 is 0.3098. The standard deviation of the death rate calculated for sample # 1 is $\frac{\sqrt{\Sigma \hat{p}_{i1}(1-\hat{p}_{i1})}}{n_1}$ $= \frac{\sqrt{0.0401+0.0430+0.0618+0.0567+0.0739}}{5} = \frac{0.5249}{5} = 0.1050$. The upper control limit based on 2 standard deviations is $0.0587 + 2 \cdot 0.1050 = 0.2687$. The observed death rate is $\frac{2}{5} = 0.4000$. Therefore, the observed death rate is significantly ($p < 0.05$) elevated relative to the expected rate. The upper control limit of sample # 2 is $0.3098 + 2 \cdot 0.1552 = 0.6208$. The observed death rate of 0.3333 is well within the control limits and pretty close to the expected value of 0.3098. Assuming that the risk adjustment is reliable, the conclusion is that the circumstances related to the two deaths in sample 1 should be carefully scrutinised. In the paper [7] where this method was originally published, the reader was cautioned not to use the equation shown in Table 6.2 to calculate wider control limits. Only 2 standard deviation limits were considered safe as assessed from simulation studies involving the author's data. The proper calculation of control limits wider than 2 standard deviations is quite complicated and beyond the scope of this book.

6.2.2   Variable Life-Adjusted Display (VLAD)

The VLAD [8] or cumulative risk-adjusted mortality chart (CRAM) [9] depicts the difference between the observed and expected cumulative mortality versus patient sample. When the outcome measure is binary, the sample size is one. For each patient the expected risk of dying (E_j) is calculated, using a risk-adjustment equation. The difference between the observed outcome (O_j) and the expected risk of dying (E_j) is calculated, and the result is added to the previous sum. We have

$$S_j = S_{j-1} + (O_j - E_j) \tag{6.2}$$

Example 6.2

Table 6.3 shows the value of Y_j for 15 consecutive patients subjected to heart surgery where $Y_j = 1$ if the patient dies within 30 days and 0 otherwise. The estimated probability of dying $(\hat{p}_{j0})$, the difference between observed outcome and expected probability of dying $(y_j - \hat{p}_{j0})$, and the cumulated sum of these differences $\Sigma(y_j - \hat{p}_{j0})$ are also shown in the table. The initial value of the sum (S_0) is usually set equal to 0. The estimated probability that the first patient dies is 0.1900. Because he/she survives we have $S_1 = S_0 + O_1 - E_1 = 0.0000 + 0.0000 - 0.1900 = -0.1900$. The estimated probability that the second patient dies is 0.2904. Because she also survives we have $S_2 = -0.1900 + (0.0000 - 0.2904) = -0.4804$. $S_3 = -0.4804 + (1.0000 - 0.4258) = 0.0938$ because the third patient dies, etc. Without risk adjustment, the expected mortality would have had a fixed value, e.g., the death rate $(\hat{p}_0)$ previously observed during a stable period. Assume $\hat{p}_0$ were 0.3333 in the actual example. Then we would have $S_1 = 0.0000 + 0.0000 - 0.3333 = -0.3333, S_2 = -0.3333 + 0.0000 - 0.3333 = -0.6666$, etc.

The VLAD chart provides valuable visual aid showing how the current performance compares to past performance. However, it is difficult to interpret since it does not specify how much variation in the plot is to be expected under acceptable performance. The charts reviewed below address this problem, but they are less intuitively appealing. Therefore, they may be used in conjunction with the VLAD chart.

6.2.3 Risk-Adjusted Probability Ratio Charts and Cusum Charts

These charts may be used to monitor binary as well as count outcome measures. For each sample a weight (W_j) is calculated and used to update a cumulative sum (S_{j-1}). This weight expresses the ratio of likelihood of

Table 6.3 The calculation of the risk-adjusted sequential probability ratio test (SPRT) using a sequence of 15 patients and the corresponding calculation when the risk is assumed to be constant and equal to 0.33.

Patient #	y_j^a	$\hat{p}_{j0}^b$	$y_j - \hat{p}_{j0}$	$\Sigma(y_j - \hat{p}_{j0})$	W_j^c	$S_{j-1} + W_j$	W_{j0}^d	$S_{j-1} + W_{j0}$
1	0	0.1900	-0.1900	-0.1900	-0.1740	-0.1740	-0.2852	-0.2852
2	0	0.2904	-0.2904	-0.4804	-0.2550	-0.4290	-0.2852	-0.5704
3	1	0.4258	0.5742	0.0938	0.3384	-0.0906	0.4080	-0.1624
4	1	0.2300	0.7700	0.8638	0.4861	0.3955	0.4080	0.2456
5	0	0.7182	-0.7182	0.1456	-0.5413	-0.1458	-0.2852	-0.0396
6	0	0.6054	-0.6054	-0.4598	-0.4734	-0.6192	-0.2852	-0.3248
7	1	0.0560	0.9440	0.4842	0.6387	0.0195	0.4080	0.0832
8	1	0.0700	0.9300	1.4142	0.6255	0.6450	0.4080	0.4912
9	1	0.0800	0.9200	2.3342	0.6162	1.2612	0.4080	0.8992
10	1	0.1937	0.8063	3.1405	0.5161	1.7773	0.4080	1.3072
11	1	0.2271	0.7729	3.9134	0.4885	2.2658	0.4080	1.7152
12	1	0.2367	0.7633	4.6767	0.4807	2.7465	0.4080	2.1232
13	1	0.2901	0.7099	5.3866	0.4384	3.1849	0.4080	2.5312
14	1	0.2904	0.7096	6.0962	0.4382	3.6231	0.4080	2.9392
15	1	0.2979	0.7021	6.7983	0.4324	4.0555	0.4080	3.3472

[a] y_j is 1 if patient # j dies and 0 otherwise.

[b] $\hat{p}_{j0}$ is the estimated probability that patient # j dies, under the assumption that the null hypothesis is true. The estimate of odds$_{j0}$ is first calculated using a logistic regression equation and the values of the patient's risk factors. Then the estimate of p_{j0} is calculated.

[c] $W_j = y_j \log(OR) - \log(1 - \hat{p}_{j0} + OR\hat{p}_{j0})$ where $OR = \frac{\hat{p}_{j1}(1-\hat{p}_{j0})}{\hat{p}_{j0}(1-\hat{p}_{j1})}$, $\hat{p}_{j0}$ is the estimated probability that patient # j dies under the null hypothesis H$_0$, and $\hat{p}_{j1}$ the estimated probability that patient # j dies under the alternative hypothesis H$_1$.

[d] W_{j0} the weight is calculated as W_j is except that the estimated probability that the patient dies is assumed to be constant and equal to 0.33.

two competing hypotheses given the observed outcome. The initial value of the sum (S_0) is usually set equal to 0.

6.2.3.1 Review of the various types of charts

All the charts originate from the sequential probability ratio test (SPRT) that was developed to choose between two hypotheses by sequential testing [10]. The SPRT chart depicts this test quantity [11]. A resetting SPRT chart is a SPRT chart that is used repeatedly to monitor a process. The risk-adjusted CUSUM chart [12] may be considered a special case of the resetting SPRT chart [13]. The calculation of the control limits of the SPRT chart is relatively straightforward. However, the calculation of the control limits of the other charts is quite complicated.

SPRT charts The SPRT chart is designed to monitor a process by accumulating the evidence in favour of each of the two competing hypotheses (H_1 and H_0) [11]. The monitoring stops when the evidence in favour of one of them is sufficiently overwhelming and this hypothesis is accepted. The cumulative sum (S_j) for this chart is equal to the previous sum plus the weight W_j. We have for the SPRT chart

$$S_j = S_{j-1} + W_j \tag{6.3}$$

The chart has two control limits, an upper one ($b > 0$) and a lower one ($a < 0$). The limits of the SPRT chart may be expressed in terms of two error rates; α and β. α is the error rate with which H_1 is accepted in favour of H_0, and β is the error rate with which H_0 is accepted in favour of H_1. The limits are calculated as follows

$$a = \log\left(\frac{\beta}{1-\alpha}\right) \tag{6.4}$$

and

$$b = \log\left(\frac{1-\beta}{\alpha}\right) \tag{6.5}$$

The chart is designed for choosing between two alternative hypotheses and not for monitoring the process beyond the time when this decision is made.

Resetting SPRT charts The resetting SPRT chart is a SPRT chart that is designed for the continued monitoring of a process [13]. This is achieved by resetting the sum to zero when the current sum crosses a control limit. If the limit is a, the monitoring is continued. Thus, H_0 is assumed to be true until it is rejected in favour of H_1. This happens when the current sum crosses the other limit, b. Then a search for a special cause is initiated. When the SPRT chart is used in this way, the meaning of the parameters β and α is lost. However, they are retained. By manipulating the values of the parameters as well as the initial value of the sum (S_0, which need not necessarily be equal to 0), charts optimised for specific purposes may be constructed [13]. However, the parameters cannot be used explicitly to calculate the control limits. Instead, a desired in-control ARL is defined, and the parameters and thereby the control limits are calculated, conditional on this ARL value. The computations involved are complicated, and the result depends on the distribution of the expected mortality risks in the data set [13].

Risk-adjusted CUSUM chart The risk-adjusted CUSUM chart [12] may be used to detect an increase or a decrease in mortality or both. In the latter case two charts are used simultaneously, one to detect an increase and one to detect a decrease in mortality. If the chart is designed to detect an increase in mortality, the sum is reset to 0 when it becomes negative. We have

$$S_j = \max\{0; S_{j-1} + W_j\} \tag{6.6}$$

If it is designed to detect a decrease in mortality, the sum is reset to 0 when it becomes positive. The cumulative sum is calculated as

$$S_j = \min\{0; S_{j-1} - W_j\} \tag{6.7}$$

It is noted that the notation of Equation (6.7) is different from that of Equation (3.7) in that a minimum value is used here. But the equations are equivalent. The calculation of control limits is complicated. Therefore, it is recommended to involve a biostatistician when designing a risk-adjusted CUSUM chart.

   We now explain how the weight used to update the cumulative sum of the above charts is actually calculated, and using an invented example we show how a SPRT chart may be calculated. The latter example also illustrates a problem, referred to as building of credit.

6.2.3.2 Calculating the probability ratio (W_j)

The weight (W_j), used to update the cumulative sum of the above charts, is a measure of the evidence of the hypothesis H_1 relative to that of the null hypothesis H_0, as documented from the observed mortality of the current patient sample. H_0 usually corresponds to performance as expected, and H_1 corresponds to a level of performance deemed importantly divergent.

Since the risk, and thereby H_0, varies from sample to sample, the alternative hypothesis cannot be expressed in terms of a fixed parameter value. Instead, the alternative hypothesis is defined in relative terms: for binary outcome measures as the ratio (OR) between the odds under H_1 and the odds under H_0, and for count outcome measures as the ratio (RR) between the expected count (λ_{j1}) under H_1 and the expected count (λ_{j0}) under H_0. The weight is calculated as the logarithm of the ratio between the probability of the observed outcome under H_1 and that under H_0. We review the calculations for each of the two outcome types.

Binary outcome Y_j is a random variable (the binary outcome measure). The probability of death $P(Y_j = 1)$, under H_1 is p_{j1}, and under H_0 it is p_{j0}. The value of the outcome measure is either $y_j = 0$ or 1. The likelihood function of $p_j = p_{j0}$, given y_j is

$$L_{0j} = P(Y_j = y_j | p_j = p_{j0}) = p_{j0}^{y_j}(1 - p_{j0})^{1-y_j}$$

Similarly, the likelihood function of $p_j = p_{j1}$, given y_j is

$$L_{1j} = P(Y_j = y_j | p_j = p_{j1}) = p_{j1}^{y_j}(1 - p_{j1})^{1-y_j}$$

W_j, the log likelihood ratio can be expressed as

$$W_j = \log\left(\frac{L_{1j}}{L_{0j}}\right) = \log\left(\frac{p_{j1}^{y_j}(1 - p_{j1})^{1-y_j}}{p_{j0}^{y_j}(1 - p_{j0})^{1-y_j}}\right)$$

$$= \log\left(\frac{\frac{p_{j1}}{p_{j0}}}{\frac{1 - p_{j1}}{1 - p_{j0}}}\right)^{y_j} + \log\left(\frac{1 - p_{j1}}{1 - p_{j0}}\right)$$

$$= y_j \log(OR) - \log(1 - p_{j0} + ORp_{j0}) \qquad (6.8)$$

where

$$OR = \frac{p_{j1}(1 - p_{j0})}{p_{j0}(1 - p_{j1})} \qquad (6.9)$$

The results can be found in [13]. To calculate W_j, we insert the y_j, which is the value of Y_j, the chosen value of OR, and the estimate of p_{j0} in Equation (6.8). To calculate p_{j1}, the chosen value of OR and the estimate of p_{j0} may be inserted in Equation (6.9) to obtain an equation in p_{j1}. Solving this, we obtain an estimate of p_{j1}.

Example 6.3

Table 6.3 shows invented data. Each sample includes a single patient. Column 1 shows the sample #, column 2 the observed outcome of an operation ($Y_j = 1$ if the patient dies and 0 if the patient survives), and column 3 shows the estimated probability of dying, calculated for each patient based on his/her risk factor values. Using the latter two values W_j (column 6) may be calculated from Equation (6.8) when the odds ratio OR is known. In the example OR has been set equal to 2. Patient # 1 survives. In this case $W_1 = 0 \cdot \log(2) - \log(1 - 0.1900 + 2 \cdot 0.1900) = -0.1740$. Patient # 3 dies. We have $W_3 = 1 \cdot \log(2) - \log(1 - 0.4258 + 2 \cdot 0.4258) = 0.3384$, etc. Column 7 shows the cumulative sum. The initial sum (not shown) is 0. $S_1 = 0 + W_1 = -0.1740$, $S_2 = -0.1740 - 0.2550 = -0.4290$, etc. W_{j0} is shown in column 8. To calculate W_{j0} it is assumed that the risk is constant and equal to that observed in the first six patients ($\frac{2}{6} = 0.33$), while the process seemed reasonably stable. W_{j0}, therefore is calculated using Equations (6.8) with a fixed value of $p_{j0} = 0.33$. The corresponding cumulative sum is shown in column 9. We calculate the control limits of a SPRT chart for $\alpha = \beta = 0.01$. We have $a = \log(\frac{\beta}{1-\alpha}) = \log(\frac{0.01}{0.99}) = -4.6000$ and $b = \log(\frac{0.99}{0.01}) = 4.6000$ (see Equations (6.4) and (6.5)). From columns 7 and 9 in Table 6.3 it appears that a decision as to which hypothesis should be preferred cannot be made neither with nor without risk adjustment.

Had we started the monitoring at patient # 7, we would have obtained the results shown in Table 6.4. This table shows the weights contributed by patients # 7 to # 15 and the cumulative sum, calculated from these weights. When we reach patient # 15, a decision can be made since the cumulative sum is $4.6747 > 4.6000$. Therefore, we decide in favour of hypothesis 1. If we inspect the probability of dying of each of the first six

Table 6.4 The calculation of the risk-adjusted sequential probability ratio test (SPRT) using a sequence of 9 patients (patients # 7–15 from Table 6.3) and the corresponding calculation when the risk is assumed to be constant and equal to 0.33.

Patient #	y_j^a	$\hat{p}_{j0}^b$	W_j^c	$S_{j-1} + W_j$	W_{j0}^d	$S_{j-1} + W_{j0}$
7	1	0.0560	0.6387	0.6387	0.4080	0.4080
8	1	0.0700	0.6255	1.2642	0.4080	0.8160
9	1	0.0800	0.6162	1.8804	0.4080	1.2240
10	1	0.1937	0.5161	2.3965	0.4080	1.6320
11	1	0.2271	0.4885	2.8850	0.4080	2.0400
12	1	0.2367	0.4807	3.3657	0.4080	2.4480
13	1	0.2901	0.4384	3.8041	0.4080	2.8560
14	1	0.2904	0.4382	4.2423	0.4080	3.2640
15	1	0.2979	0.4324	4.6747	0.4080	3.6720

[a] y_j is 1 if patient # j dies and 0 otherwise.
[b] $\hat{p}_{j0}$ is the estimated probability that patient # j dies, under the assumption that the null hypothesis is true. The estimate of odds$_{j0}$ is first calculated using a logistic regression equation and the values of the patient's risk factors. Then the estimate of p_{j0} is calculated.
[c] $W_j = y_j \log(OR) - \log(1 - \hat{p}_{j0} + OR\hat{p}_{j0})$ where $OR = \frac{\hat{p}_{j1}(1-\hat{p}_{j0})}{\hat{p}_{j0}(1-\hat{p}_{j1})}$, $\hat{p}_{j0}$ is the estimated probability that patient # j dies under the null hypothesis H_0, and $\hat{p}_{j1}$ the estimated probability that patient # j dies under the alternative hypothesis H_1.
[d] W_{j0} the weight is calculated as W_j is except that under H_0, the estimated probability that the patient dies is assumed to be constant and equal to 0.33.

patients (see Table 6.3), we find the reason why the conclusion differed in the two situations. Patients # 5 and # 6 both had a high probability of dying. But they survived, indicating that the surgeon was very skilled or very lucky. Therefore, the corresponding weights are both relatively low (-0.5413 and -0.4734). Consequently, some credit is being accumulated, and the cumulative sum attains a low value (-0.6192) for patient # 6. From patient # 7 and on, the mortality clearly rises. However, the credit of -0.6192 prevents the cumulative sum from crossing the upper limit of 4.6000. The fact that the cumulative sum in Table 6.4 does not cross the limit when the probability of H_0 is fixed at 0.33 is explained by the estimated probabilities of patients # 7 and # 8 (see Table 6.4). They both have a rather low probability of dying. Loosing patients #7 and # 8, therefore, is heavily penalised in the presence of risk adjustment, but far less so without risk adjustment.

Count outcome When the outcome measure is a count, H_0 states that the expected count is equal to the count (λ_{j0}) predicted from the risk model, and H_1 states that

$$\lambda_{j1} = RR \cdot \lambda_{j0} \tag{6.10}$$

where RR is a constant, usually equal to 2, and λ_{j1} is the expected count under H_1. Let y_j be the observed count of adverse events, and Y_j be the corresponding random variable. Since it is assumed that Y_j follows a Poisson distribution, it follows that the likelihood function of $\lambda_j = \lambda_{j0}$, given y_j is

$$L_{0j} = P(Y_j = y_j | \lambda_j = \lambda_{j0}) = \frac{\lambda_{j0}^{y_j}}{y_j!} e^{-\lambda_{j0}} \tag{6.11}$$

Similarly, the likelihood function of $\lambda_j = \lambda_{j1}$, given y_j is

$$L_{1j} = P(Y_j = y_j | \lambda_j = \lambda_{j1}) = \frac{\lambda_{j1}^{y_j}}{y_j!} e^{-\lambda_{j1}} \tag{6.12}$$

W_j, the log likelihood ratio can be expresses as follows

$$W_j = \log\left(\frac{L_{1j}}{L_{0j}}\right) = \log\left(\left(\frac{\lambda_{j1}}{\lambda_{j0}}\right)^{y_j} e^{-(\lambda_{j1} - \lambda_{j0})}\right)$$

$$= y_j \log\left(\frac{\lambda_{j1}}{\lambda_{j0}}\right) - (\lambda_{j1} - \lambda_{j0})$$

$$= y_j \log(RR) - \lambda_{j0}(RR - 1) \tag{6.13}$$

where $RR = \frac{\lambda_{j1}}{\lambda_{j0}}$. See results in [13]. To obtain W_j, we insert the chosen value of RR and the estimated value of λ_{j0} in Equation (6.13).

6.3   COMMENTS

In this and previous chapters we have only reviewed the most commonly used control charts. But there are other charts [14–17], e.g., the set chart. The set chart is a generalisation of the type of chart that was used to monitor the number of days (X) between two infections in Example 2.6. The X chart used in Example 2.6 signals an alarm when X becomes smaller than a specified limit (k). By contrast, the set chart allows this limit to be crossed a preset number of times (n) before it signals an alarm. The idea is that for specified in-control ARL, k and n may be chosen so that the out-of-control ARL is minimised [16, 17]. In the risk-adjusted version of the set chart, the number of patients surviving replaces the number of days. Furthermore, the difference between the patients in terms of their risk of dying is taken into account. It is not quite clear which of the two charts is better; the set chart or the CUSUM chart. For further details of the risk-adjusted set chart see the paper by Grigg and Farewell [18].

The reader should be aware that a number of problems related to risk-adjusted control charts are still unresolved [19]. The ratio between observed and expected number of outcomes does not necessarily follow a Gaussian distribution, and the results are not necessarily independent. Furthermore, the observed number of events within a heterogeneous population (comprising patients with different risks) is not a simple random variable. These issues require further research.

REFERENCES

[1] Eisenstein EL, and Bethea CF. The use of patient mix-adjusted control charts to compare in-hospital costs of care. Health Care Manage Sci 1999; 2:193–8.
[2] Hart MK, Robertson JW, Hart RF, and Lee KY. Application of variables control charts to risk-adjust time-ordered healthcare data. Qual Manage Health Care 2003; 13:99-119.
[3] Hollenbeak CS. Functional form and risk adjustment of hospital costs: Bayesian analysis of a Box-Cox random coefficients model. Stat Med 2005; 24:3005–18.
[4] Parsonnet V, Dean D, and Bernstein AD. A method of uniform stratification of risks for evaluating the results of surgery in acquired adult heart disease. Circulation 1989; 19(1 suppl): 1–12.
[5] Steiner SH, Cook RJ, Farewell VT, and Treasure T. Monitoring surgical performance using risk-adjusted cumulative sum charts. Biostatistics 2000; 1: 441–52.
[6] Grigg O, and Farewell V. An overview of risk-adjusted charts. J Roy Stat Soc A 2004; 167:523–39.
[7] Cook DA, Steiner SH, Cook RJ, Farewell VT, and Morton AP. Monitoring the evolutionary process of quality: risk-adjusted charting to track outcomes in intensive care. Crit Care Med 2003; 31:1676–82.
[8] Lovegrove J, Valencia 0, Treasure T, Sherlaw-Johnson C, and Gallivan S. Monitoring the results of cardiac surgery by variable life-adjusted display. Lancet 1997; 350:1128–30.
[9] Poloniecki J, Valencia O, and Littlejohns P. Cumulative risk adjusted mortality chart for detecting changes in death rate: observational study of heart surgery. Br Med J 1998; 316:1697–1700.
[10] Wald A. Sequential tests of statistical hypotheses. Ann Math Stat 1945; 16: 117–86.
[11] Spiegelhalter DJ, Grigg O, Kinsman R, and Treasure T. Risk-adjusted sequential probability ratio tests (sprts) for monitoring risk-adjusted outcomes. Int J Qual Health Care 2003; 15:7-13.
[12] Steiner SH, Cook RJ, Farewell VT, and Treasure T. Monitoring surgical performance using risk-adjusted cumulative sum charts. Biostatistics 2000; 1: 441–52.

[13] Grigg O, Farewell VT, and Spiegelhalter DJ. Use of risk-adjusted CUSUM and RSPRT charts for monitoring in medical contexts. Stat Methods Med Res 2003; 12:147–70.

[14] Ismail NA, Pettitt AN, and Webster RA. 'Online' monitoring and retrospective analysis of hospital outcomes based on a scan statistic. Stat Med 2003; 22:2861–76.

[15] Naus J, and Wallenstein S. Temporal surveillance using scan statistics. Stat Med 2006; 25:311–24.

[16] Chen RA. Surveillance system for congenital malformations. J Am Stat Assoc 1978; 73:323–27.

[17] Gallus G, Mandelli C, Marchi M, and Radaelli G. On surveillance methods for congenital malformations. Stat Med 1986; 5:565–71.

[18] Grigg O, and Farewell VT. A risk-adjusted sets method for monitoring adverse medical outcomes. Stat Med 2004; 23:1593–1602.

[19] Benneyan JC, and Borgman AD. Risk-adjusted sequential probability ratio tests and longitudinal surveillance methods. Int J Qual Health Care 2003; 15:5–6.

7

Risk-Adjusted Comparison of Healthcare Providers

Variability of outcome measure results among healthcare providers may be due to random variation, lack of standardisation of the outcome measure, data errors, differences in the case-mix, and differences in the quality of care. The same is true for the results measured within the same provider at different times. A healthcare provider may be a hospital, a hospital department, a private practice, a physician, etc. Comparative assessment of the results of treatment and care either requires that the patient groups are comparable in terms of measured and unmeasured risk factors, or if this cannot be accomplished, that the case-mix differences are adjusted for, by using statistical manipulation of the data. In Section 7.1, we discuss how comparable patient groups may be produced experimentally. In Section 7.2, we explain how one may attempt to adjust observational data for case-mix differences, using the tools presented in Chapter 5. Interpretation of the results obtained using the latter approach is fraught with problems. This is discussed in Section 7.3. Because it has become mandatory in many countries to publicise outcome comparisons across hospitals and practices, the pros and cons of this approach are discussed in Section 7.4.

7.1 EXPERIMENTAL ADJUSTMENT

If patients are assigned at random to one of several healthcare providers whose quality of care we want to compare, the case mix of the resulting patient groups will be balanced, except for differences that occur for random reasons. Therefore, standard statistical techniques are valid, and the interpretation of the results is straightforward. The benefit of randomisation may be improved if important risk factors for the outcome in question are known and measured in the patients prior to the randomisation. Sampling at random is then done from each stratum, a priori defined by the risk factor(s). Therefore, the distribution of the strata across the healthcare units to be compared may be perfectly balanced. The actual randomisation and the conduct of the experiments require careful planning if allocation bias is to be evaded. A review of the planning and conduct of randomised controlled experiments is beyond the scope of this book. The interested reader is referred to the book by Pocock [1], which provides an excellent introduction to this topic.

There is no doubt that randomisation of patients to the healthcare units to be compared is the proper scientific approach. The problem, of course, is that in general it is quite complicated and expensive to conduct a randomised clinical trial.

Example 7.1

An excellent solution to this problem is to organise the healthcare system so that the infrastructure allows randomised clinical trials to be conducted at a modest extra cost. This is the approach taken at the Metro-Health Medical Center in Cleveland Ohio [2]. They organised ongoing random assignment of patients and providers to three teams or 'firms'. Department faculty was randomised to the firms after stratifying by subspecialty. The director of department of medicine is the head of the three firms, but each firm has its own director and separate inpatient unit and outpatient practice area staffed by nonrotating personnel.

Examples where this approach has been used include, e.g., a trial of interdisciplinary rounds on the inpatient medical wards conducted at the MetroHealth Center [3]. Prior to the trial, a task force examined the existing process of care using flow charts. They found that the interdisciplinary interactions were minimal and episodic and nonemergent orders were written throughout the day, making the nursing and pharmacy workloads unpredictable. The traditional rounds included physicians only, charts were left at the nursing station, and structured multidisciplinary rounds were held only once a week. By contrast, the interdisciplinary rounds included physicians, patient-care coordinator, pharmacist, nutritionist, and social worker. Orders were written during these rounds, and the patient charts were taken to the rounds. There was no weekly multidisciplinary round since it proved unnecessary. The effects of introducing interdisciplinary rounds were a significant reduction of the average length of stay from 6.06 to 5.46 days and of the average charges per patient from 8090 to 6681 dollars.

Example 7.2

In a study that lasted from January 2000 until July 2002, Ferguson *et al.* randomised 359 academic and nonacademic hospitals, participating in the Society of Thoracic Surgeons National Cardiac Database [4], to a control arm or to one of two intervention groups that used continuous quality improvement (CQI) (see Section 7.4 for a formal definition). The hospitals treated 267 917 patients using coronary artery bypass graft (CABG) surgery during the study period. The CQI was designed to increase the use of two process of care measures, one in each intervention group. They included preoperative β-blockade and internal mammary artery (IMA) grafting. The CQI comprised information about the measure, including a call to action to a physician leader, educational products, and periodic, nationally benchmarked, feedback. Preoperative β-blockade and IMA grafting both increased nationally during the study period. For preoperative β-blockade, the increase was significantly higher in the intervention group (3.6 % increase in the control arm versus 7.3 % increase in the intervention arm). A similar, but insignificant trend was observed for the IMA grafting. Therefore, the effect of introducing CQI increased the use of β-blockade above a value that may be explained by the national trend.

7.2 STATISTICAL RISK ADJUSTMENT OF OBSERVATIONAL DATA

When data do not originate from a randomised experiment, adjustment may be effected using statistical methods. They are all based on the belief that either (1) all risk factors of major importance for the prediction of a specified outcome are known and measurable or (2) some of them are, and the distributions of the remaining ones are balanced across all patient groups that are to be compared. The values of the known risk factors are measured in each patient and used to risk-adjust the patient groups. The two most widely used methods will be presented. One is based on the identification of one or more groups of patients where the distributions of the risk factors are balanced between the subgroups belonging to different healthcare providers. The other is based on a modelling of the relation between the risk factor(s) and the outcome.

7.2.1 Identification of Risk Factor Balanced Groups

The least complicated method of identifying groups where the distributions of risk factors are balanced between the subgroups belonging to different healthcare providers is to use stratification. However, as will be explained below, it is usually necessary to apply a more complicated method, namely the propensity score method.

7.2.1.1 Stratification

A simple method for risk adjustment is to divide the patients into groups (strata) with the same risk characteristics. For instance, if sex and diabetes are the risk factors, the patients are divided into four groups, female nondiabetics, female diabetics, male nondiabetics, and male diabetics. Comparisons between the healthcare providers are performed within each of these strata. The overall difference between the healthcare providers is calculated by computing a weighted average of the within strata estimates of the differences [5]. This approach is best used when the number of risk factors is quite limited, i.e., one or two. When the number of risk factors is large, it becomes impractical or impossible to use this method because the number of strata mushrooms.

7.2.1.2 Propensity score methodology

Propensity score methodology, introduced by Rosenbaum and Rubin [6], addresses the above problem by reducing the entire collection of background variables to a single composite characteristic, the propensity score. The propensity score is a patient's probability of being assigned to one of two alternative 'interventions', as determined by that patient's covariate values. In the present context, 'intervention' is the patient's assignment to one of two healthcare providers. It may be shown that for a group of patients having the same propensity score the subgroups of patients assigned to different providers will have the same joint distribution in all the covariates that were used to estimate the propensity score. An informal proof of this is given in [7]. This theoretical result is exploited as follows: a logistic regression equation is calculated using the risk factors observed in the patients whose propensity scores we want to calculate. The dependent variable is the odds of being assigned to 'intervention 1' and the independent variables are the risk factors (or covariates) that we want to adjust for. Using this equation, the odds of being assigned to the intervention group are estimated in each patient. The patient's propensity score is finally calculated from the odds, using Equation (5.16). After the propensity scores have been estimated, the following three approaches are possible:

Method 1 All patient pairs, one from each intervention group, with estimated propensity scores that are sufficiently alike are found and the comparison between the two intervention groups is confined to these patients. 'Being sufficiently alike' may be defined in various ways [8]. Patients for whom no match can be found are eliminated from the analysis. To avoid bias, this matching of pairs ought to be done without knowledge of the outcome in question.

Method 2 The patients are sorted in ascending order according to the value of the estimated propensity score. The data set is then divided into strata defined by the value of the score. For instance, five equally sized groups may be formed. Comparisons are made within each stratum, and the overall treatment effect is estimated as a weighted average of the within-strata estimates of the intervention effect.

Method 3 A binary variable, the provider variable, is defined. It is equal to 1 if the patient was assigned to provider # 1 and 0 otherwise. A regression is then performed. The outcome (for continuous outcome measures) or the odds of outcome (for binary outcome measures) is the dependent variable. The estimated propensity score and the provider variable are the independent variables. This model will estimate the relationship between the estimated propensity score and the outcome (or odds of outcome). Therefore, the effect of the propensity score and thereby of the risk factors used to estimate the score are adjusted for when the effect of the provider on the outcome measure is estimated.

The larger a data set is, the more successful the propensity score method will be in adjusting for the risk factors [7].

Example 7.3

Oo *et al.* [9] used the abovementioned regression technique when they compared the effect of training surgeons on the in-hospital coronary artery bypass graft (CABG) surgery mortality and morbidity. The odds

ratio of in-hospital CABG surgery mortality between trainee-led operations and consultant-led ones was 0.37 with a 95 % confidence interval
(CI) of 0.15–0.90. The trainee-led operations had a significantly better
outcome than the consultant-led ones since 1.00 was not included in the
95 % CI. However, the patients operated on by the consultants were
generally more difficult and high-risk patients. Therefore, Oo *et al.* used
the propensity-score technique. In this analysis 'intervention 1' corresponds to a trainee-led operation and 'intervention 2' to a consultant-led
operation. The propensity score is the probability that a patient will be
subjected to an operation led by a trainee, as predicted using the risk
factors that we want to adjust for. The outcome measure is in-hospital
death following operation.

Using logistic regression, Oo *et al.* estimated the relationship between
independent risk factors and the propensity for a trainee-led CABG and
obtained the following equation

$$
\begin{aligned}
\text{logit(propensity score)} = {} & -1.5674 + 0.0190\,(\text{age}) \\
& -0.1711(\text{female sex}) \\
& -0.0359\,(\text{body mass index}) \\
& -0.4906\,(\text{ejection fraction30\%}) \\
& -0.799\,(\text{three vessel disease}) \\
& +0.4260\,(\text{previous myocardial infarction}) \\
& -1.8272\,(\text{prior cardiac surgery}) \\
& -0.1163\,(\text{Euro Score})
\end{aligned}
$$

$$(7.1)$$

where age, body mass index (BMI), and the Euro Score [10] are continuous variables, and the rest are binary indicator variables that are
equal to 1 if the statement indicated by the indicator name is true.

We will estimate the propensity score of a 55-year-old female with
BMI of 25, ejection fraction 30 %, without three-vessel disease, without
previous acute myocardial infarction, without prior cardiac surgery, and
with a Euro score of 4. We have

$$
\begin{aligned}
\text{logit(propensity score)} = {} & -1.5674 + 0.0190 \cdot 55 - 0.1711 \cdot 1 \\
& -0.0359 \cdot 25 - 0.4906 \cdot 1 \\
& -0.799 \cdot 0 + 0.4260 \cdot 0 \\
& -1.8272 \cdot 0 - 0.1163 \cdot 4 = -2.5468.
\end{aligned}
$$

The odds are $e^{-2.5468} = 0.0783$. Using Equation (5.16), the propensity score may be estimated as $\frac{0.0783}{1+0.0783} = 0.073$. Therefore, the estimated probability that this patient will be subjected to a trainee-led operation is 0.073.

Due to the limited sample size, the authors preferred method 3 described above. To compare the odds of in-hospital mortality between trainee-led and consultant-led operations they estimated a logistic regression equation of the type (the equation was not reported), $\text{logit}(p) = a + b_1$ propensity score $+ b_2$ 'trainee'. 'Trainee' is a binary variable that is equal to 1 if the operation is led by a trainee and 0 if led by a consultant; p is the probability of in-hospital death. The authors found an odds ratio for in-hospital mortality between trainee-led operations and consultant-led ones of 0.65 with a 95 % CI of 0.26 to 1.64. Since the 95 % CI included 1.00, the odds ratio did not differ significantly from 1. Therefore, these results suggest that the quality of the trainee led operations do not differ significantly from that of the consultant-led ones.

We used an example of method 3 because in our opinion this is the least intuitively obvious method and it is the most popular one.

However, the success of the application of a propensity score methodology ought to be assessed by its ability to balance the distributions of the covariates between the treatment groups to be compared. The distributions should be similar with insignificant differences between the treatment groups. Method 3 mentioned above suffers from the disadvantage that this assessment cannot be done. Therefore, methods 1 and 2 may be preferred applications.

An important difference between the method used in Section 7.2.2 and the propensity score method is that the requirements for a logistic regression model [11] described in Section 5.5 in Chapter 5 do not necessarily apply when the regression model is used to estimate the propensity scores. For instance, if the regression equation provides a complete discrimination between the intervention groups, the method is useless. The reason is that it is not possible to find pairs of patients with matching propensity scores belonging to different intervention groups. The test of a good propensity score model is whether it adequately balances the risk factors. Therefore, the model need not necessarily be parsimonious and easy to understand. So, it may include numerous covariates (including those with statistically insignificant coefficients) and interactions and nonlinear terms [12]. In fact, the role of the previously recommended criteria (see Section 5.5 in Chapter 5) for logistic regression modelling in the estimation of useful propensity scores is poorly understood [13].

Often it is necessary to compare more than two healthcare providers. However, the propensity score methodology may be modified to allow adjustment when more than two healthcare providers are compared [14, 7].

One may speculate that the propensity score methodology may be preferable to a modelling of the relation between risk factors and outcome (see Section 7.2.2). The reason is that it is possible to directly verify whether a given application of the propensity score methodology has been successful or not. Therefore, the risk adjustment is not done blindly, so to speak. However, systematic reviews of the literature, where propensity score methods and regression models (see Section 7.2.2) have both been used, showed that similar results were obtained using the two methods [12, 15]. The authors noted that one explanation might be that the propensity score method had not been well implemented in most studies.

The propensity score method is not some magical method that is guaranteed to remove all kinds of bias between the intervention groups compared. For instance, propensity score methods cannot control for unknown, unmeasured, or imperfectly measured variables that affect outcome. Therefore, residual systematic bias cannot be excluded.

7.2.2 Modelling the Relation between Risk Factor(s) and Outcome

When the relation between risk factors and outcome is modelled, we examine if the type of relationship between measured risk factors and the outcome (or some function of the outcome) is linear. If this is not the case, we devise suitable transformations of the variables and/or include additional derived variables to adjust for important interactions and/or non-linear relationships between the original variables, hoping that a linear relationship emerges. The resulting linear regression model is used to separate the variation of the results of the outcome measure between patients within healthcare provider from the corresponding variation between healthcare providers. In this way variation caused by case-mix differences between the providers is separated from that caused by differences in the quality of care and treatment between the providers.

The results of such an analysis may depend heavily on the statistical model used and the risk factors selected [16–19]. In Chapter 5 we reviewed various statistical models. It was recommended to include the provider effect directly in the model either as a fixed effect (see Equation

(5.19)) or preferably as a random effect (see Equations (5.20) and (5.21)).

The results may either be reported using a direct standardisation or an indirect standardisation [20]. Under direct standardisation [21], a standard population is used to estimate how many events a hospital may experience if its case mix were similar to that of the standard population, but its quality of care unchanged. It is assumed that the outcome measure is binary. Under indirect standardisation, a standard population is used to estimate the expected number of events at each hospital if its quality of care were similar to that of the standard population, but its case mix was unchanged. The latter approach is the one generally chosen, but it has been criticised [22]. Since binary outcome measures are the most commonly used and hierarchical models seem to have certain advantages over more conventional models, we will explain how the indirectly standardised mortality rates are computed using a random intercept hierarchical, generalised linear model [23].

The model is given by

$$\text{logit}(Y_{ij} = 1 | X_{ij}, \beta_{0j}, \beta_1) = \text{logit}(p_{ij}) = \beta_{0j} + \beta_1 X_{ij} + \varepsilon_{ij} \quad (7.2)$$

For simplicity there is only one risk factor. β_1 is a fixed effect independent of patient and hospital, and X_{ij} is the risk factor measured in patient # i who is treated at hospital # j. β_{0j} is a random hospital effect that is assumed to follow a normal distribution with mean μ and variance τ^2. Thus, μ is the mean of the population of hospitals and τ^2 is a measure of the individual hospitals' variation relative to this mean. Y_{ij} is 1 if the patient experiences the event (say death within 30 days following CABG surgery) and 0 otherwise. Using a computer program the parameters of Equation (7.2) are estimated. The estimated odds of patient # i in hospital # j are $e^{\hat{\beta}_{0j} + \hat{\beta}_1 x_{ij}}$ and the corresponding estimated probability is

$$\hat{p}_{ij} = \frac{e^{\hat{\beta}_{0j} + \hat{\beta}_1 x_{ij}}}{1 + e^{\hat{\beta}_{0j} + \hat{\beta}_1 x_{ij}}} \quad (7.3)$$

(see Equation (5.16)).

The smoothed, hospital specific mortality rate for hospital number # j, adjusted for case mix is given by

$$\frac{1}{n_j} \sum_{i=1}^{n_j} \frac{e^{\hat{\beta}_{0j} + \hat{\beta}_1 x_{ij}}}{1 + e^{\hat{\beta}_{0j} + \hat{\beta}_1 x_{ij}}} = O_j \quad (7.4)$$

where n_j is the number of patients treated at hospital # j. The expected probability of death for patient # i (if treated at an average hospital in the region examined) is

$$\frac{e^{\hat{\mu}+\hat{\beta}_1 x_{ij}}}{1 + e^{\hat{\mu}+\hat{\beta}_1 x_{ij}}} \tag{7.5}$$

where the average intercept $(\hat{\mu})$ for all providers is used. The corresponding expected mortality rate is

$$E_j = \frac{1}{n_j} \sum_{i=1}^{n_j} \frac{e^{\hat{\mu}+\hat{\beta}_1 x_{ij}}}{1 + e^{\hat{\mu}+\hat{\beta}_1 x_{ij}}} \tag{7.6}$$

The standardised mortality incidence rate (RAM_j) is

$$RAM_j = \frac{O_j \cdot MR}{E_j} \tag{7.7}$$

where MR is the unadjusted mortality rate for the whole region. The RAM_j with credible probability interval may be compared to the region average mortality rate. If the latter is not included in the credible probability interval, the hospital is an outlying hospital and the reason for this should be investigated. Reference to software and technical details may be found in [23]. It is recommended that a professional statistician with experience in mixed models analyses performs the calculations. In the above model hospital characteristics such as teaching status, volume, etc. were not incorporated. However, this is certainly possible [24] and may provide additional valuable information. If this is done, the reference population should still be the whole region. If comparisons are done within each specific hospital category, the effect of significant hospital characteristics such as teaching status and volume will be masked, and the consumers may be misled.

7.3 PERILS OF RISK ADJUSTING OBSERVATIONAL DATA

Statistical risk adjustment of observational data has the potential for generating results that may be very misleading. Therefore, great care should be taken when applying the results. We present the results of some simulation experiments to illustrate one simple and intuitively obvious mechanism whereby misleading results may be produced. However, first we will explain the principles of the simulation experiments.

Assume that we have two types of patients, type-1 and type-2. The probability that a type-1 patient dies during a specified and properly administered surgical procedure is 0.1, and the probability that a type-2 patient dies is 0.3. If these probabilities are constant over time, the surgical procedure is in a state of statistical control. This means that its quality is stable.

The behaviour of such a process over time may be simulated. Assume we wanted to simulate the experience of 1000 consecutive type-1 patients who were subjected to the surgical procedure. To do so, we perform 1000 independent experiments, each simulating the experience of one patient. Each experiment consists of a random draw of one ball from an urn containing 10 % red balls and 90 % white balls, simulating the 10 % probability of death during operation. If we wanted to simulate the experiences of a mixture of type-1 and type-2 patients, we would use two urns, one for type-1 patients containing 10 % red balls and another for type-2 patients, containing 30 % red balls. Instead of drawing balls from urns the experiments may be done using a standard statistical package on a computer.

Example 7.4

Imagine two hospitals both receiving patients belonging to the same well-defined clinical entity and suffering from the same severe disease that requires major surgery. Assume that the same surgical procedure is used in both hospitals and that two patient factors influence these patients' risk of dying during operation: the presence of a specific genetic trait (R_1: 1 if the factor is present, otherwise 0) and the presence of infection of the organ to be operated on (R_2: 1 if present, otherwise 0). Patients with neither risk factor present have a 0.1 probability of dying during the procedure, regardless of which hospital they are admitted to. For patients with one factor present the probability is 0.3, and for those with both factors present it is 0.6.

We now conduct a simulation experiment based on the above mentioned assumptions, simulating the experience of 2000 patients admitted to the two hospitals. To study the effect of case mix we vary the patient case mix between the hospitals. We examine the effect of risk adjustment when both risk factors are known and when only risk factor 2 is known.

Table 7.1 shows for each of the above two hospitals the case mix of 1000 patients admitted to the hospital and the results of the simulation experiments. These results have been analysed under the assumption that both risk factors are known to the medical community (columns 5 and 6)

Table 7.1 The results of a simulation study where the probability of death during a surgical procedure as a function of two risk factors (R_1: presence of a genetic trait and R_2: presence of infection of the organ operated on) was simulated. The probability of death, for given risk factor combination, is the same in the two hospitals but the case mix differs between the hospitals.

Hospital[a]	Genetic trait[b] R_1	Infected organ[c] R_2	Simulated model[d]	Result of simulation[e] Mortality[g]	n (no. dead)[h]	Genetic trait assumed unknown[f] Mortality[i]	n (no. dead)[i]
1	No	No	$p = 0.1$	0.060	100(6)	0.227	300(68)
	Yes	No	$p = 0.3$	0.310	200(62)		
	No	Yes	$p = 0.3$	0.300	200(60)	0.496	700(347)
	Yes	Yes	$p = 0.6$	0.574	500(287)		
2	No	No	$p = 0.1$	0.096	700(67)	0.131	840(110)
	Yes	No	$p = 0.3$	0.307	140(43)		
	No	Yes	$p = 0.3$	0.233	120(28)	0.381	160(61)
	Yes	Yes	$p = 0.6$	0.825	40(33)		

[a] It is assumed that the quality of treatment and care is the same at the two hospitals.
[b] The presence of the genetic trait influences the probability of death (see parameters of simulation model in column 4).
[c] The presence of infection of the organ operated on influences the probability of death (see parameters of simulation model in column 4).
[d] The parameter value of the simulation model generating the data. For instance when the genetic trait is present and the organ is infected the probability of death is 0.6.
[e] Column 5 and 6 show the result of the simulation for each combination of risk factors in each hospital.
[f] Column 7 and 8 show how the results would have been classified had the information of the genetic trait been unknown to the medical community. For instance the results of the two first sets of experiments would have been pooled and classified as data from patients without organ infection, etc.
[g] The mortality observed in each of the 8 sets of simulation experiments. When compared to the value in column 4 one may appreciate the effect of the random variation.
[h] n is the number of independent simulations done per experiment. n has been varied between the hospitals to imitate differences between the case mixes of the two hospitals. No. dead is the number of fatal outcomes occurring during the n simulations.
[i] Using the same data that were generated by the simulation. For given value of 'infected organ' and given hospital the data have been pooled imitating the situation where the risk factor 'genetic trait' is unknown to the medical community.

and under the assumption that only one is known (columns 7 and 8). For example, row 1 of hospital # 1 shows the simulated probability of death in column 4. It is 0.1 because the patients of this category do not have any of the two risk factors present (see columns 2 and 3). The result of the simulation of 100 patients' experience is that six patients died (column 6). Row 2 of hospital # 1 shows the corresponding results for patients with risk factor 1 present and risk factor 2 absent. Here the simulated probability of death is 0.3 and the result of the simulation that 62 of the 200 patients died giving a simulated death rate of 0.310. Columns 7 and 8 show how the results would have been interpreted had risk factor 1 been unknown to the medical community. Now, the two types of patients cannot be distinguished and we calculate the mortality for patients with risk factor 2 absent as $\frac{68}{300}= 0.227$, etc.

The overall mortality rates (hospital # 1: 0.415 and hospital # 2: 0.171) differ significantly between hospitals. However, we need to adjust for the difference in case mix. To do so, we perform a regression of risk factors and the hospital effect on logit(p_{ij}) where p_{ij} is the probability that patient # i, treated at hospital # j, dies. There are only two hospitals; we are only interested in these hospitals, and the experiments were independent of each other. Therefore, we use a fixed-effect model. The independent variables include R_1, R_2, and H_1 (1 if the patient is treated at hospital # 1 and 0 if treated at hospital # 2). We have the model

$$\text{logit}(p_{ij}) = \alpha + \beta_1 R_{1i} + \beta_2 R_{2i} + \delta_1 H_1 + \varepsilon_{ij}.$$

Table 7.2 shows the result of the logistic regression analysis. The coefficients of both risk factors are highly significantly different from 0 while that of the hospital effect is not. This is no surprise to us because we

Table 7.2   The estimated coefficients of two logistic regressions of hospital $(H_1)^a$ and risk factors^b (R_1 and R_2) on logit(p), where p is the probability of dying during an operation. In the first regression analysis^c both risk factors were known. In the second analysis^d it was assumed that only one of the risk factors (factor 2) was known, imitating the situation where an important risk factor is unknown to the medical community.

	All risk factors known				One risk factor assumed unknown			
Parameter	Estimate	SE^e	p^f	Estimated odds ratio^g	Estimate	SE	p	Estimated odds ratio
β_2	1.30	0.127	0.00005	3.67	1.29	0.123	0.00005	3.63
δ_1	−0.139	0.144	0.34	0.871	0.57	0.125	0.00005	1.77
β_1	1.46	0.127	0.00005	4.32	Factor assumed unknown			

^{a} H_1 is a binary variable that is 1 if the patient was operated on at hospital # 1 and 0 if the patient was operated on at hospital # 2.
^{b} Risk factor 1 (R_1), 'presence of genetic trait'. $R_1 = 1$ if trait is present, otherwise 0. Risk factor 2 (R_2), 'presence of infection in organ operated on'. $R_2 = 1$ if infection is present, otherwise 0.
^{c} logit(p) $= \alpha + \beta_1 R_1 + \beta_2 R_2 + \delta_1 H_1 = -2.23 + 1.46 R_1 + 1.30 R_2 - 0.139 H_1$ (For simplicity indices referring to patient # and hospital # have been omitted).
^{d} logit(p) $= \alpha + \beta_2 R_2 + \delta_1 H_1 = -1.86 + 1.29 R_1 + 0.57 H_1$.
^{e} SE = standard error of estimate.
^{f} p-value.
^{g} e^{estimate}. For example, for the parameter β_2 we have $e^{1.30} = 3.67$.

conducted the experiment so that the hospitals only differed in terms of their case-mixes.

Table 7.1 (columns 7 and 8) shows how the data resulting from the simulation would have been classified had the genetic trait been unknown. Patients with both risk factors present would not be distinguishable from patients with only risk factor 2 present and patients with only risk factor 1 present would be classified as low risk patients. The logistic regression model, therefore, becomes

$$\text{logit}(p_{ij}) = \alpha + \beta_2 R_{2i} + \delta_1 H_1 + \varepsilon_{ij}.$$

Table 7.2 shows that now the hospital coefficient is significantly different from 0 (p-value $= 0.00005$) implying that the mortality rate of hospital # 1 is higher than that of hospital # 2 even if we adjust for the observable case-mix differences. Thus, the presence of an unknown or unmeasured significant risk factor (here R_1) may bias the comparisons between healthcare providers.

Following a simulation of random assignment of the patients to the two hospitals, 1009 patients, of whom 316 died, were assigned to hospital # 1, while 991, of whom 300 died, were assigned to hospital # 2. The two mortality rates were 0.313 and 0.303, i.e., almost identical, showing unambiguously that the two hospitals do not differ importantly.

Empirical studies [25] have demonstrated that statistical adjustment of observational data may fail to remove the main part of bias and occasionally increases systematic bias. This may result from omitted or unknown risk factors (as illustrated in the above example), misspecification of continuous variables (inappropriate conversion to binary variables or failure to recognise nonlinear relationships), misclassification caused by the use of poor proxies for the proper covariate, measurement errors, and within-patient instability in covariate (e.g., because of circadian rhythms). We refer the reader to a very thorough and interesting discussion in the paper by Deeks *et al.* [25].

As a minimum we suggest that the following six points be considered when statistical risk adjustment of observational data is attempted

1. Data are first presented without adjustment.
2. Continuous variables, e.g., age or weight are not transformed into binary variables since this throws away information and increases the likelihood of improper model specification.

3. The assumptions of the model building such as linearity, etc. (see Chapter 5 Section 5.5) are checked. Where the propensity score methodology is used, the balance of risk factor distributions between treatment groups must be verified.
4. When appropriate a hierarchical model is used.
5. The variation not accounted for by the risk adjustment model is measured and reported.
6. As a rule of thumb, observational data are considered hypothesis-generating material and treated accordingly, and very explicitly presented as such. That is, the results should be presented as needing experimental verification before any conclusions may be drawn.

Considering the problematic nature of observational data, the publicising of such data may give rise to some concern. In the following section we address this topic.

7.4   PUBLIC REPORT CARDS

There is an increasing demand for accountability. As a response to this demand, it has become mandatory in many jurisdictions to release public report cards, comparing outcomes across hospitals or practice groups. This raises the questions: what are the potential advantages and dangers related to the publicising of report cards showing outcome data, and how should the medical community react?

The proponents of the publicising of report cards argue that it encourages quality improvement through market forces. The opponents recommend using the principles of continuous quality improvement (CQI). The principles of CQI are based on confidentiality. It uses benchmarking, determination of 'best practice', and collaborative education among physicians. Shahian *et al.* published a thorough and penetrating analysis of these problems in relation to cardiac surgery report cards in an excellent paper from 2001 [26]. It offers a good illustration of the problems and controversies that may be related to the publicising of outcome data. They reviewed the literature on the release of report cards in the New York State. Here the names and risk-adjusted mortality rates of individual surgeons are publicised statewide. Between 1989 and 1992, 27 surgeons with less than 50 cases a year and with risk-adjusted mortality rate 2.5 to 5 times the state average stopped performing CABG surgery, either voluntarily or because of restriction of hospital privileges [27, 28]. Shahian *et al.* admit that the magnitude of improvement in the New York State CABG surgery mortality may have exceeded the nationwide improvement. However, they suggest that it may be a result of quality improvement initiatives undertaken by individual hospitals. This contention is supported by a study [29], showing that the northern New England area that had used an aggressive, but completely confidential CQI approach, was the only region that had a mortality reduction comparable to that of the New York State (see also [30]).

Publicising performance data may have adverse effects. They include, for example, avoidance of high-risk cases. The reason for this is that surgeons are concerned that risk adjustment provides inadequate protection from the higher mortality rates that they are experiencing when operating on high-risk patients. Although there is conflicting objective evidence regarding avoidance of high-risk CABG surgery patients, many surgeons perceive that accepting such cases may jeopardise their reputations and careers (see, e.g., [31]). Another concern has been that the existence of public report cards may result in so-called gaming that may be responsible for apparent improvements in risk-adjusted mortalities. Gaming includes excess reporting (up-coding) of preoperative co-morbidities, change of the operative procedure of high-risk patients from a reported category to a nonreported category, and transfer of critically ill patients to extended care facility before their anticipated death because mortalities occurring in these facilities are not reported. It seems likely that some degree of up-coding has occurred as a result of public report cards. The frequency of change of operative procedure is difficult to quantify. But the problem does exist and has been described (see, e.g., [32]). The last problem (change of risk adjusted mortality by transfer of critically ill postoperative patients) may be avoided by collecting outcome data at a fixed time regardless of where the patient has been transferred.

Several precautions may be taken to prevent some of the above potential problems. During the planning and implementation of report cards, there is a need for constructive, nonadversarial collaboration between clinicians, statisticians, and regulators [33]. Preferably the database to be used for the report card should be national or statewide and supported by the relevant professional societies. Not the least, education of the media is important to facilitate fair and dispassionate press coverage.

REFERENCES

[1] Pocock SJ. Clinical Trials – A Practical Approach. Wiley and Sons Ltd Chichester, 2002.

[2] Cebul RD. Randomized, controlled trials using the metro firm system. Med Care 1991; 29(suppl):JS9–JS18.

[3] Curley C, McEachern JE, and Speroff T. A firm trial of interdisciplinary rounds on the inpatients medical wards: an intervention designed using continuous quality improvement. Med Care 1998; 36(suppl):AS4–AS12.

[4] Ferguson TB, Peterson ED, Coombs LP, Eiken MC, Carey ML, Grover FL, and DeLong ER. Use of continuous improvement to increase use of process measures in patients undergoing coronary artery bypass graft surgery. JAMA 2003; 290:49–56.

[5] Yanagawa T, Fujii Y, and Mastuoka H. Environ Health Perspect 1994; 102(suppl):57–60.

[6] Rosenbaum PR, and Rubin DB. The central role of the propensity score in observational studies for causal effects. Biometrika 1983; 70:41–55.

[7] Rubin DB. Estimating causal effects from large data sets using propensity scores. Ann Intern Med 1997; 127:757–63.

[8] D'Agostino RB, Jr. Tutorial in biostatistics: propensity score methods for bias reduction in the comparison of a treatment to a non-randomized control group. Stat Med 1998; 17:2265–81.

[9] Oo AT, Grayson AD, and Rashid A. Effect of training on outcomes following coronary artery bypass graft surgery. Eur J Cardiothorac Surg 2004; 25:591–6.

[10] Nashef SA, Roques F, Michel P, Gauducheau E, Lemeshow S, and Salamon R. European system for cardiac operative risk evaluation (EuroSCORE). Eur J Cardiothorac Surg 1999; 16:9–13.

[11] Bagley SC, White H, and Golomb BA. Logistic regression in the medical literature: standards for use and reporting, with particular attention to one medical domain. J Clin Epidemiol 2001; 54:979–85.

[12] Shah BR, Laupacis A, Hux JE, and Austin PC. Propensity score methods gave similar results to traditional regression modelling in observational studies: a systematic review. J Clin Epidemiol 2005; 58:550–9.

[13] Weitzen S, Lapane KL, Toledano AY, Hume AL, and Mor V. Principles for modelling propensity scores in medical research: a systematic literature review. Pharmacoepidem Dr S 2004; 13:841–53.

[14] Huang IC, Frangakis C, Dominici F, Diettc GB, and Wu AW. Application of a propensity score approach for risk adjustment in profiling multiple physician groups on asthma. Health Serv Res 2005; 40:253–78.

[15] Sturmer T, Joshi M, Glynn RJ, Avorn J, Rothman KJ, and Schneeweiss S. A review of the application of propensity score methods yielded increasing use, advantages in specific settings, but not substantially different estimates compared with conventional multivariable methods. J Clin Epidemiol 2006; 59:437–47.

[16] Krumholz HM. Mathematical models and the assessment of performance in cardiology. Circulation 1999; 99:2067–9.

[17] Naftel DC. Do different investigators sometimes produce different multivariable equations from the same data? J Thorac Cardiovasc Surg 1994; 107:1528–9.

[18] Poses RM, McClish DK, Smith WR, Huber EC, Clemo FLW, Schmitt BP, Alexander D, Racht EM, and Colenda CC. Result of report cards for patients with congestive

heart failure depend on the method used to adjust for severity. Ann Intern Med 2000; 133:10–20.

[19] Spiegelhalter DJ. Probabilistic prediction in patient management and clinical trials. Stat Med 1986; 5:421–33.

[20] Romano PS. Peer group benchmarks are not appropriate for health care quality report cards. Am Heart J 2004; 148:921–3.

[21] Christiansen CL, and Morris CN. Improving the statistical approach to health care provider profiling. Ann Intern Med 1997; 127:764–8.

[22] Rixom A. Performance league tables. BMJ 2002; 325:177–8.

[23] Shahian DM, Torchiana DF, Shemin RJ, Rawn JD, and Normand SL. Massachusetts cardiac surgery report card: implications of statistical methodology. Ann Thorac Surg 2005; 80:2106–13.

[24] Austin PC, Alter DA, Anderson GM, and Tu JV. Impact of choice of benchmark on the conclusions of hospital report cards. Am Heart J 2004; 148:1041–6.

[25] Deeks JJ, Dinnes J, D'Amico R, Sowden AJ, Sakarovitch C, Song F, Petticrew M, and Altman DG. Evaluating non-randomised intervention studies. Health Technol Assess 2003; 7:1–173.

[26] Shahian DM, Normand SL, Torchiana DF, Lewis SM, Pastore JO, Kuntz RE, and Dreyer PI. Cardiac surgery report cards: comprehensive review and statistical critique [Review]. Ann Thorac Surg 2001; 72:2155–68.

[27] Chassin MR, Hannan EL, and DeBuono BA. Benefits and hazards of reporting medical outcomes publicly. N Engl J Med 1996; 334:394–8.

[28] Hannan EI, Siu AL, Kumar D, Kilburn H, and Chassin MR. The decline in coronary artery bypass graft surgery mortality in New York: the role of surgeon volume. JAMA 1995; 273:209–13.

[29] Peterson ED, DeLong ER, Jollis JG, Muhlbaier LH, and Mark DB. The effects of New York's bypass surgery provider profiling on access to care and patient outcomes in the elderly. J Am Coll Cardiol 1998; 32:993–9.

[30] Guru V, Fremes SE, Naylor CD, Austin PC, Shrive FM, Ghali WA, and Tu JV. Public versus private institutional performances reporting: what is mandatory for quality improvement? Am Heart J 2006; 152:573–8.

[31] Schneider EC, Epstein AM. Influence of cardiac-surgery performance reports on referral practices and access to care: a survey of cardiovascular specialists. N Engl J Med 1996; 335:251–6.

[32] Carey JS, Dziuban SW, Arom KV, Cimochowski GE, Plume SK, and Grover FL. Quality improvement in thoracic surgery, Bull Am Coll Surg 1998; 83:24–9.

[33] Shahian DM, Torchiana DF, and Normand SL. Implementation of a cardiac surgery report card: lessons from the Massachusetts experience Ann Thorac Surg 2005; 80:1146–50.

Part III

Learning and Quality Assessment

8

Learning Curves

When a new nonpharmacological clinical procedure is introduced, e.g., a new surgical procedure, it is sometimes argued that it is unfair to evaluate it because enough experience in using the technique has not yet been gathered. When this has been accomplished, the technique may be so well established that it is too late to evaluate it. It is then argued that it would be unethical to have a control group of patients who will not benefit from the procedure. However, the quality of a clinical procedure (e.g., a minimally invasive surgical procedure) that is carried out repeatedly by the same person may be measured using an appropriate quantity.

The measured quality of a new clinical procedure usually improves over time, but at a declining rate. Gradually it then reaches a stable value of quality (the asymptote). The expected time course of the process variable used to characterise the procedure is referred to as a learning curve. In this chapter we present methods that may be used to monitor the quality of a nonpharmacological procedure from the time when it is introduced and until sufficient experience in using the procedure has been gained. In this way the above dilemma may be resolved. When the assessment of the procedure is initiated without delay, it will have two advantages: (1) the minimum experience necessary to master the technique may be assessed, and (2) the asymptote may be compared to the quality of already established alternative procedures. In the latter comparison one must remember the risks of comparing apples with oranges (i.e., comparing different case mixes, see Chapter 7).

Statistical Development of Quality in Medicine P. Winkel and N. F. Zhang
© 2007 John Wiley & Sons, Ltd

8.1 ASSESSING A SINGLE LEARNING CURVE

Before a learning curve can be described, a measure of the quality of the procedure should be selected. The value of this quantity is measured each time the procedure is performed by the same person. The procedures performed are numbered according to their chronological order, and the number is referred to as the sequence number. Next, one checks if a trend (a learning effect) can be detected. If this is the case, one proceeds to characterise the learning curve. The measure of quality is usually either continuous or binary. An example of a continuous one that is quite popular is the time it takes to perform a surgical procedure (the operating time). But other continuous measures, e.g., the length of stay at hospital of a patient subsequent to having been subjected to a surgical procedure, are also possible. An example of a binary one is the presence versus absence of intra-operative complication. We show how to approach the data analysis in each of these two cases.

8.1.1 Continuous Measure of Quality

To analyse learning curve data, a scatter diagram of the quality measure versus sequence number is first drawn. To get a clearer picture, various types of data treatment, such as the calculation of a moving average may be used [1]. If a trend may be discerned visually, one proceeds and examines if a statistically significant learning effect can be demonstrated. Sorting the observations in ascending order, according to their sequence numbers may achieve this. They are then divided into three or four approximately equally sized groups, and a statistical test is used to test if the group means differ significantly and if a time trend may be detected. Once a significant trend is detected, the learning curve is established. In Example 5.2 we demonstrated the principles that may be applied. The following example is adapted from a study by Ramsay et al. [2].

Example 8.1

They measured the operating time of 190 consecutive laparoscopic fundoplication procedures (an operation of the stomach) performed by a single surgeon. We have read their data from the figure in their paper.

Figure 8.1 depicts the operating time as a function of the sequence number of the operation. It seems that there is a slight trend, so that the

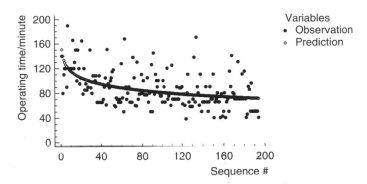

Figure 8.1 The operating time of laparoscopic fundoplication operations (surgery of the stomach) performed by the same surgeon depicted as a function of the sequence number of the operation (filled circles). We have read the data from a figure in a paper by Ramsay *et al.* [2]. The function: operating time/minute = 158.25 (sequence #)$^{-0.146}$, that was fitted to the data, is also shown on the figure (open circles).

operating time declines with increasing sequence number. When a moving average algorithm is applied to the data (result not shown), this impression gets clearer. Ramsay *et al.* proceeded to demonstrate the presence of a trend as described above and then tried to fit various functions to their data.

The three best types of functions are shown in Table 8.1. We applied the power law to the data of Figure 8.1 (see Example 5.2). The estimated parameters were $a = 158.25$ and $b = -0.146$. The function is depicted in Figure 8.1.

Ramsay *et al.* found that the power law explained 20 %, i.e., the R^2 of $Y = aX^b$ was 20 %. This, of course, is much less than was the case in the idealised Example 5.2.

Table 8.1 Three types of functions that have been used to predict the quality of a nonpharmacological procedure (Y) as a function of its sequence number (X); a and b are the parameters of the functions (see paper by Ramsay *et al.* [2]).

Type of curve	Equation
Power law	$Y = a \cdot X^b$
Logarithmic	$Y = a \cdot \ln(X) + b$
Log-linear	$Y = e^{(a + Xb)}$

8.1.2 Binary Measure of Quality

From a statistical point of view, a continuous quality indicator is ideal since it is relatively easy to analyse. However, from a clinical point of view a binary indicator may often be more appropriate. The operating time may not necessarily be a good proxy of quality. It may just be a proxy of the experience gained in using the same type of quality. The problem is that the event studied when using a binary measure may be very rare. The cumulative sum (CUSUM) may be used as an exploratory technique to discern a trend when the quality measure is binary. Example 8.2 offers an illustration.

Example 8.2

Table 8.2 shows an invented data set. For each of 20 surgical procedures, the occurrence of intra-operative complication ('failure') has been coded

Table 8.2 Cumulative sum (CUSUM) of deviations between observed outcome and expected probability of failure measured in each of 20 consecutive surgical procedures. The data are invented. Failure is defined as the occurrence of intra-operative complication.

Procedure #	Observed outcome[a] (A)	Expected probability of failure (B)	Deviation (A − B)	CUSUM
1	1.0	0.3	0.7	0.7
2	0.0	0.3	−0.3	0.4
3	1.0	0.3	0.7	1.1
4	1.0	0.3	0.7	1.8
5	0.0	0.3	−0.3	1.5
6	0.0	0.3	−0.3	1.2
7	1.0	0.3	0.7	1.9
8	0.0	0.3	−0.3	1.6
9	1.0	0.3	0.7	2.3
10	0.0	0.3	−0.3	2.0
11	0.0	0.3	−0.3	1.7
12	0.0	0.3	−0.3	1.4
13	1.0	0.3	0.7	2.1
14	0.0	0.3	−0.3	1.8
15	0.0	0.3	−0.3	1.5
16	0.0	0.3	−0.3	1.2
17	0.0	0.3	−0.3	0.9
18	0.0	0.3	−0.3	0.6
19	1.0	0.3	0.7	1.3
20	0.0	0.3	−0.3	1.0

[a] Occurrence of complication is coded as 1 and lack of occurrence of complication is coded as 0.

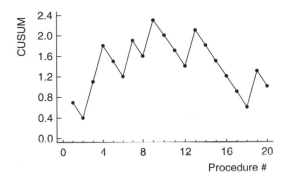

Figure 8.2 The cumulative sum (CUSUM) of the deviations between the observed binary outcome and the expected (0.3) probability of failure of surgical procedures. Failure is defined as the occurrence of intra-operative complication.

as 1 and lack of occurrence as 0. A proficiency level of 70 % is assumed implying that complication should not occur in more than 30 % of the operations. Therefore, the expected probability of 'failure' is 0.3 (column 3). In column 4 the observed outcome minus the expected one is shown. The CUSUM, shown in column 5, is the cumulative sum of these deviations. Initially (observations 1 to 4) the failure rate (the average of the failure codes) is larger than the target (0.3). Then it equals it (observation 5 to 14), and finally it goes below the target rate (observation 15 to 20).

Figure 8.2 depicts the CUSUM curve. As long as the failure rate is larger than the target, the curve rises. While it is equal to the expected value, it is flat (not as a pancake), and when the rate goes below the target, it declines. This is a typical pattern when a learning effect is present.

This technique has been used in the literature. The procedure number reached when the CUSUM begins to decline is defined as the number of procedures necessary to attain an acceptable performance.

Once a learning pattern is demonstrated, the data may be ordered in ascending sequence number and divided into three to four equally sized groups. It may then be tested if a significant learning effect is present. If this is the case, logistic regression may be applied to estimate a learning curve, as illustrated in the following example.

Example 8.3

From the figures in Ramsay *et al*. [2], we read the results of a binary outcome variable, defining the appearance of one or more complications

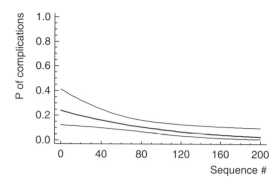

Figure 8.3 Probability of the occurrence of complication during a laparoscopic fundoplication operation (surgery of the stomach) as a function of the operation's sequence number (bold line). The function was estimated using logistic regression analysis. The 95 % confidence interval of the function is also depicted in the figure (thin lines).

during the operation measured in each of the first 190 laparoscopic fundoplication operations made by the same surgeon. Using these data, we performed a logistic regression of sequence # of operation on logit(p), where p is the probability of complication. The following equation was derived as the result of the analysis

$$\widehat{\text{logit}}(p) = -1.162 - 0.012 \text{ sequence \#} \tag{8.1}$$

Therefore, $\frac{p}{1-p}$ is equal to $e^{-(1.162+0.012 \text{ sequence \#})}$. We may now estimate the probability that intra-operative complication will occur during operation # 191. The odds of complication is $e^{-(1.162+0.012\cdot191)}$, and according to Equation (5.16) the estimated probability of complication is

$$\frac{e^{-(1.162+0.012\cdot191)}}{1+e^{-(1.162+0.012\cdot191)}} = \frac{0.0316}{1+0.0316} = 0.0306.$$

Figure 8.3 depicts the estimated probability as a function of the procedure sequence number computed by the *Statgraphics* program. The 95 % confidence interval band, calculated by the program, is also depicted in the figure.

8.1.3 Case-Mix Adjustment

The variation relative to the predicted line may include variation that can be ascribed to differences between the patients who are operated on, in terms of sex, age, concomitant diseases, etc. As shown in Chapter 5, one may attempt to compensate for this case-mix effect by including the significant factors as covariates in the logistic regression. Ramsay *et al.* included a number of patient-related covariates in the logistic function, but found that none of them were significantly associated with the dependent variable. However, when they included various covariates in the power law function relating log(operating time/minute) to log(sequence #), the patient's age did influence the learning curve significantly. When age was included, 24 % of the variation was explained as compared to 19 % when only the sequence # was included. Still, this is far from 100 %. Case mix, sometimes, complicates the assessment of learning curves [2]. As a physician gets more experienced, he/she may get a relatively large proportion of the severe cases. Therefore his/her quality may appear to decline over time (see Example 7.3).

8.2   ASSESSING MULTIPLE LEARNING CURVES

If the learning curves of a specified procedure differ significantly between physicians, the curve of each individual physician should be estimated. If not, the data may be pooled to obtain a single curve, e.g., characterising a single institution. Ramsay *et al.* studied multiple operators [2] in a prospective study of laparoscopic cholecystectomy using the power law model after logarithmic transformation, as explained in Example 5.2. Using a mixed model (see Chapter 5), they demonstrated that a model might describe the data where the 10 operators may be described as a random sample from a population of operators, with individual starting levels (a in Equation (5.2)) and learning rates (b in Equation (5.2)) deviating at random from the corresponding population mean values. They found that starting levels and learning rates differed significantly between operators and explained 15 % of the total variability. Seven percent of the within operator variability was explained by the operator's learning curve as opposed to 20 % for the laparoscopic fundoplication procedure. When they included sex, gall bladder rupture, and presence of inflammation of the gallbladder in their model, they found that these covariates contributed significantly to the total variability.

The mixed model (see Chapter 5) used by them allows the disentangling of the proportion of total variability that can be attributed to true variation in rates of learning from surgeon to surgeon from that proportion, which can be attributed to random variation between patients within surgeons. Similar techniques may be applied if the quality measure is a binary variable [3]. However, as explained in Chapter 7, risk adjustment of observational data is fraught with problems. Clearly, a design where the patients are assigned at random to the operators is preferable. However, in practice, it may be difficult, sometimes impossible to carry out such an experiment.

From the study by Ramsay *et al.*, we may learn that learning curves may differ between technologies and between physicians, and not least that variation due to case mix may play a role. We also learn that a large proportion of the variability cannot be explained. This may be ascribed to case-mix variation that has gone unrecognised. Of course, these results cannot necessarily be generalised.

8.3   FACTORS AFFECTING LEARNING CURVES

There are reasons to believe that the institutions where the procedures are performed may impact the learning curves [4]. Table 8.3 shows the factors that may affect individual learning curves at various levels of the hierarchy of a healthcare organisation. At the first level, we have the patient. Here, individual patient characteristics and the clinical characteristics of the population of patients undergoing the procedure may influence the learning curve. At the second level, we have the physician whose attitude, natural abilities, capacity for acquiring new skills, and previous experience may have an influence. At the third level is the institution. The institution can impact on the learning curve through the organisation of facilities, financial means, and the experience and type of people included in the team supporting the physician.

Table 8.3   Factors that may influence a learning curve at various levels of a healthcare hierarchy.

Level of hierarchy	Factors
Institution	Organization, finances, quality of supporting team.
Physician	Natural skills and experience.
Patient	Individual patient characteristics, type of clinical target population.

8.4 LEARNING CURVES AND RANDOMISED CLINICAL TRIALS

When the infrastructure of a healthcare organisation allows it, randomised clinical trials may be economically and practically feasible to conduct. In that case, one may compare the impact of a new procedure, e.g., a surgical one, on the quality of treatment, by comparing it to the quality of an older and well-established procedure. In a randomised trial, variation over time in case mix and other factors that may impact the results of the procedures compared are accounted for because the patients are allocated at random to interventions within each of the participating institutions. Therefore, the effect of these factors is balanced between the intervention groups, in that any difference is only random. However, the effect of the improvement in skill in performing the new procedure that occurs over time will not be neutralised by the randomisation. Therefore, this may obscure the results unless the effect is measured and taken into account when the quality is compared between the procedures.

Figure 8.4 illustrates the problem. It depicts invented data showing the monthly mortality rates of two patient groups, A and B as a function of the duration of a randomised trial with two arms designed to compare the mortality rate of a new surgical procedure (arm A) to that of an older well-established surgical procedure (arm B). It is obvious from the figure that the new procedure is better than the old one since the mortality rate of arm A is below that of arm B once the two mortality rates are stable. It

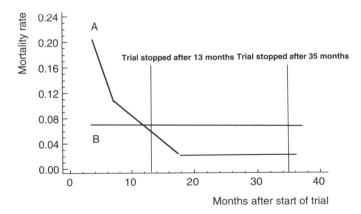

Figure 8.4 The mortality rate of two patient groups, A and B, depicted as a function of the duration of a randomised clinical trial comparing two interventions, a new surgical procedure (group A) and one currently used (group B). The data are invented.

is also obvious that a learning effect is present for the new procedure. If the trial were to be stopped after 13 months, a comparison between the mortality rates of the two groups would imply that the old procedure is superior to the new one. If it were to be stopped after 35 months, the result would indicate the opposite to be the case.

REFERENCES

[1] Kendall M. Time-series. Hafner Press, New York, 1976.
[2] Ramsay CR, Grant AM, Wallace SA, Garthwaite PH, Monk AF, and Russell IT. Statistical assessment of the learning curves of health technologies. Health Technol Assess 2001; 5:1–79.
[3] Cook JA, Ramsay CR, and Fayers P. Statistical evaluation of learning curve effects in surgical trials. Clin Trials 2004; 1:421–7.
[4] Bull C, Yates R, Sarkar D, Deanfield J, and deLeval M. Scientific, ethical, and logistical considerations in introducing a new operation: a retrospective cohort study from paediatric cardiac surgery. BMJ 2000; 320:1168–73.

9

Assessing the Quality of Clinical Processes

To assess the quality of clinical processes on a routine basis, an information system, integrated in the existing clinical information system and designed for the measurement of clinical quality, must be in place. The lack of proper, well-functioning information technology systems has been a major obstacle to the development of routine clinical quality control and assessment. Once the data are available, they must be subjected to a statistical analysis, the outcome of which is the assessment of the quality.

In this chapter, we discuss the data processing aspect and describe how to benchmark processes in statistical control. When several healthcare providers are benchmarked, it is assumed that they are in statistical control, in the same state. That is, the variation between providers can be explained by the within-provider variation over time. This latter assumption may be assessed, using a so-called funnel chart. However, it is the exception rather than the rule that the assumption is fulfilled. It is emphasised that the actions that are to be taken, when lack of statistical control has been discovered, should be prespecified and considered at the design stage of the monitoring system. Sometimes an excessive number of providers are outside the control limits. This phenomenon is referred to as overdispersion. In this situation various approaches are possible.

9.1 DATA PROCESSING REQUIREMENT

To monitor and assess the quality of clinical processes *on a routine basis*, there are certain design considerations that must be addressed, before it becomes cost effective. The data collection, storage, and processing must be highly automated and well integrated in existing clinical data-processing systems. When designing a system, its future use must be anticipated. If the data are only used for the physician or to select physicians whose practices should be the subject of a closer review, some imprecision could be tolerated. However, if the purpose is to make critical, professional decisions, e.g., recertification, the data should be clinically meaningful and very reliable [1]. Therefore, a statement of the purpose of a reporting system is necessary. To ensure that the data will be meaningful, the database should be collected specifically for the performance assessment [1]. Documentation of the experience of physicians and institutions, e.g., number of procedures performed, specialty, location, etc., may be important indicators of quality. Therefore, these data should be available. Traceability of the scientific evidence upon which the system is based is a key consideration. Definitions and algorithms used when collecting and presenting the data as well as reference to sources from which they originate must be documented and supplemented with a logbook, specifying the periods of their usage.

Recently a set of guiding principles and operational steps for the development of functional information systems in health care has been published [2]. The author of the guidelines envisioned an integrated system where healthcare delivery groups generate data for internal operations in a way that makes it possible to combine these data into high-level reports on accountability. We review these principles and operational steps.

9.1.1 Guiding Principles for the Development of an Information System

A functional information system should include four key elements: (1) single-point data collection at point of entry, (2) the prerequisite for combining data for multiple purposes, (3) the prerequisite for securing privacy and confidentiality of patient records, and (4) audit standards.

9.1.1.1 Single-Point data collection at point of entry

The aim of this is to eliminate redundancy. Furthermore, the data will usually be more accurate and complete than data entered at secondary time points. For instance, when the blood pressure is measured in a patient, it is entered directly into the clinical information system.

9.1.1.2 Prerequisite for combining data for multiple purposes

Data may be used, not only for local purposes such as direction of patient care, summary reports for an individual clinician or care delivery team, but also for aggregate reporting across conditions (e.g., all surgical procedures) or across groups of providers or geographical regions within the same clinical measure. Aggregate reporting relies on four concepts: classes of outcome, a common metric, an analytical method, and patient registries (with master index systems to create accurate denominators).

Classes of outcome Classes of outcome may include (1) *medical* (complications, result of therapy etc., from the clinician's perspective), (2) *patient functional status* (patient's perspective on treatment effects), (3) *service* (dimensions of the patient-clinician relationship, e.g., access and convenience), (4) *cost* (expenditures associated with medical care processes). They may be combined with three additional measures: *patient stratification* (includes factors that cannot be controlled by the provider, but influence outcomes, e.g., demographics), *appropriateness* (includes factors used to determine if an intervention is appropriate, e.g., failure of maximal medical therapy to control angina), and key *process factors* that determine outcome (e.g., timely administration of medicine).

Common metrics Appropriate common metrics for these major outcome classes must be agreed on, to produce meaningful and consistent aggregate reports across regions or nations. For example, the indications, that determine the appropriateness of a surgical procedure for a particular patient, are tailored to a specific clinical scenario. All surgical procedures might be combined using the common metric *appropriateness*. The report would then contain the proportion of all surgical procedures that were performed for clinically appropriate reasons.

As another example, consider the fingerprinting of a particular clinical condition. A list of common defects should be prepared. However, functional definitions should also be prepared to stage each defect. To allow diverse outcomes to be classified on a common metric, a staging system must be developed, so that summary performance scores can be reported. An example is the staging system, originally suggested by the US Center for Disease Control and Prevention [2]. This includes four stages: stage 1, event without risk of long-term harm occurred. No intervention. Stage 2, event without risk of long-term harm occurred. Intervention was undertaken to speed recovery. Stage 3, event occurred, patient was at risk for long-term harm; but intervention prevented that harm from occurring. Stage 4, the patient suffered a long-term injury (minor, major, or death). Using this system defects could be summarised across conditions and organisational units.

Agreement on analytical methods   Data system design should include agreement on analytical methods, used to combine data across care delivery groupings and clinical conditions.

Patient registries   Such registries are a means of maintaining the data across a care delivery group or a geographical area. They deliver the proper denominators, needed to generate rate of performances (e.g., all diabetic patients in a practice within a defined time period).

9.1.1.3   Prerequisite for securing confidentiality of patient records

The third principle relates to the protection of the patients' privacy and the confidentiality of the clinical data pertaining to the patient. Ideally (in our opinion) one should strike a proper balance between, on one side, the need to consult the patient and conceal sensitive clinical information for those not directly involved in the clinical decision making, and on the other side the need to control the costs and secure the availability of timely and important clinical information for those involved in the clinical decision making. Clearly, the current and anticipated legislation on patient confidentiality should be taken into consideration when an information system is constructed.

9.1.1.4   Audit standards

The final principle is to secure an appropriate auditing of the system. Data system audits should attempt to limit the role of the measurement system as a major source of variation in reported results. This implies that the completeness and accuracy of data are controlled. The completeness of data should be checked at the population level (are all patients present and accounted for?) and on the individual case level (are all data fields present and accounted for?). The audit of the accuracy of data includes a content analysis to assess whether standard coding definitions are consistently followed. To secure an impartial audit, each measurement set developed should include explicit standards for concurrent data audits, and the auditors must be completely independent of the care delivery group they review.

9.1.2   Functional Steps in Designing a Data System

The functional steps in designing a data system on a regional or national basis are based on the key concept that condition-specific sections are added to the data base that grows in breadth and depth over time. To generate individual modules within such a system, the following procedure is recommended. One starts with the desired end result and works backwards to the front-line data collection and data flow. The steps include focusing on a high-priority clinical process, development of a conceptual model, generation of a list of reports, determination of data elements based on these reports, identification of already automated data, and testing the system. Once the test is successful, the system is implemented.

9.1.2.1   Focus on high-priority clinical processes

Clinical processes may be divided into: (1) clinical conditions (outpatient/primary care and inpatient/specialty care); (2) clinical support services (laboratory, etc.); (3) service quality; and (4) administrative support processes. The first step is to assess these various clinical processes to select those that will have the greatest effect and then invest in them.

9.1.2.2   Development of a conceptual model

The next step is to develop a conceptual model of the selected process. Such models provide a context for individual tasks and link them together into a co-ordinated workflow. One approach would be to start

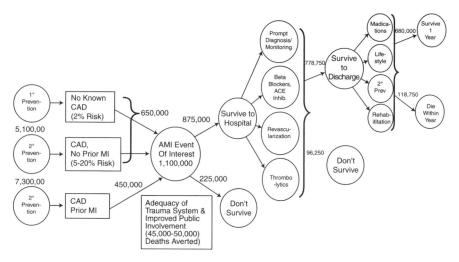

Figure 9.1 Clinical logic for acute myocardial infarction. Reproduced with permission from McGlynn EA. Selecting common measures of quality and system performance. Med Care 2003; 41(suppl):I-39–I-47.

with a conceptual flow diagram. Here one takes advantage of the natural hierarchy found in real processes. One starts with a simple flow diagram of the whole clinical process. Then those steps that hold the most potential for improvement or most strongly control the outcome are identified. These steps are expanded to form a second more detailed layer. One continues in this way until a decision layer is reached. The result is a traditional decision flowchart.

Figure 9.1 from the study by McGlynn [3] shows a conceptual clinical flow diagram for acute myocardial infarction (AMI). Based on evidence from the literature one may estimate the proportions of the deaths that are preventable through improved care. Doing this, underscores the importance of primary and secondary prevention of AMI. Therefore, one continues to expand this part of the flow diagram.

9.1.2.3   Generation of list of reports

The third step is to generate a list of reports and test their utility. Each box in the flow diagram above the decision level is examined, and it is determined which report should routinely be generated to track performance and outcomes. Model reports containing real data or simulated data are circulated to those who are expected to use them, and the questions are asked: (1) is the information useful? (2) Is it presented where it is needed for the decision maker? (3) How often should the report be generated?

9.1.2.4   Determination of data elements based on report list

The fourth step is to use the report list to determine the data elements required routinely to produce information for decision makers. A coding manual is produced and developed into coding sheets where a coding sheet is defined as a shorthand-coding manual for practical data entry use. This scheme could be pilot tested.

9.1.2.5   Identification of already automated data

The fifth step is to identify those data that are already automated and those that have to be obtained in the course of care delivery. Then the data acquisition strategy is designed in collaboration with those on the frontline where the data are generated.

9.1.2.6   Testing

The sixth step is to test the final reporting system, before full-scale implementation is attempted. This is quite important. Experience in real data systems has shown that shortcuts during the planning and testing phases are likely to lead to increased costs and decreased functionality.

9.1.2.7   Implementation

When the system has been successfully tested, it is implemented.

9.2   BENCHMARKING OF PROCESSES IN STATISTICAL CONTROL

When meaningful data are readily available, the clinical processes may be characterised and their quality assessed, using various statistical techniques. Assessment of clinical quality may be achieved using external standards (benchmarking). If possible, a benchmark should be based on professional judgement. However, often it is necessary to resort to an average, such as a national average. If this is done it will also be important to assess how this national average compares with averages of other nations.

A healthcare unit may be a surgeon, a practitioner, a hospital, etc. Direct comparison between comparable healthcare units tends to focus the attention on outlying healthcare units. The lack of a common standard, based on which the organisation as such could be evaluated, makes it difficult to assess the results. If the general standard is high, outlying units below the average quality may be quite acceptable. On the other hand, if the general standard is very low, outlying units with above average quality may be quite unacceptable [4].

A necessary prerequisite for a meaningful assessment of the quality is statistical control of the processes examined. In Chapter 2, we characterised an asthma patient, using a control chart of her peak expiratory flow rate (PEFR). Initially the PEFR was in statistical control and, therefore, predictable. In fact, it could be predicted that the patient could easily develop an asthma attack. Thus, her state was clinically unsatisfactory. Therefore, the treatment was changed so that the PEFR stabilised at a more normal level. The example illustrates that although statistical control has nothing to do with quality, it is necessary to attain statistical control to be able to assess the quality of the process; in the example, the treatment of the patient. If a process is not in statistical control, it is unpredictable, and consequently, in principle, its quality cannot be assessed.

9.2.1   Benchmarking of a Single Healthcare Provider

To assess the quality of a process using external standards, the following steps are necessary: (0) the quality requirements are specified; (1) the process is brought in statistical control; (2) its quality is measured; and (3) the quality is assessed by comparing the measured quality to the requirements. If the quality does not meet the requirements, the process is modified and steps 1 through 3 are repeated, etc. This is the classical approach used in industrial quality control and development.

9.2.1.1   Defining the quality requirements

In industry, the quality requirements are often expressed as a nominal value, characterising the products of the highest quality and an upper (USL) and lower (LSL) specification limit. The USL is the highest and the LSL is the lowest value that the process variable may assume for the product to be acceptable. An example is the production of nuts (to be used for a screw). Let the process variable be the internal diameter of the nut. The nominal value depends on what the nuts are to be used for. It seems logical for this example to choose USL and LSL so that they are located symmetrically around this value. Sometimes, industrial quality requirements are expressed by a single specification limit, i.e., a USL or an LSL, that the values of the process variable should be far below or above, respectively.

Example 9.1

In asthma patients the lowest acceptable value of the peak expiratory flow rate may be calculated. For the patient presented in Example 2.7, this value was 188 l/min. Therefore, in this case the quality requirement is expressed as an LSL, i.e., 188 l/min.

In the scientific biomedical literature, recommended therapeutic procedures and corresponding clinical target populations, expected outcomes, and frequencies of adverse effects, are published continuously. Meta-analyses of these publications provide useful syntheses and summaries that may be used as external standards in the assessment of the measured quality of clinical processes. However, the use of published performance data, e.g., expected mortality rates, as external standards may not be that simple because it may be difficult to determine if the patient population is comparable to patient datasets published. However, monitoring the frequency of the proper usage of treatments according to published evidence is certainly possible.

9.2.1.2   Characterising the process

Before the quality of a process can be compared to quality requirements, it has to be measured, i.e., the distribution of the process variable must be characterised. The mean of the process variable is a measure of the typical product produced by the process. The capability of a process refers to its capability to produce uniform products, and the standard deviation of the process variable is a measure of this capability. The smaller the standard deviation is, the more uniform are the products.

In industry, the process capability is often measured as six times the standard deviation of the process variable. Therefore, it makes sense to define the natural tolerance limits of a process as the mean, $\mu \pm 3$ standard deviations (3σ) of the process variable. If the latter follows a Gaussian distribution, 99.73 % of its values are expected to fall within the natural tolerance limits. A more general definition of the natural tolerance limits would be an interval that excludes 0.135 %, which is $\frac{100\% - 99.73\%}{2}$ of the most extreme high values and the 0.135 % of the most extreme low ones. In the following, the equations will be derived under the assumption that the process variable is continuous and follows a Gaussian distribution. It is also assumed that a USL is larger and an LSL is smaller than the mean.

9.2.1.3 Relating process to quality requirements

Figure 9.2 shows the distribution of a process variable. The quality requirement is defined as a USL. The fraction of unacceptable products is depicted as the area (A) of the distribution that lies to the right of the USL. 'Upper' is the upper natural tolerance limit, and 'Lower' is the lower one. The area to the right of 'Upper' includes 0.135 % of the distribution. In this example, the fraction of undesirable products exceeds 0.135 % (A includes the 0.135 % area, lying to the right of 'Upper'). If USL and 'Upper' were identical, the fraction of unacceptable products would be 0.135 %. If USL were located to the right of 'Upper', the fraction would be less than 0.135 %. For an LSL the same type of

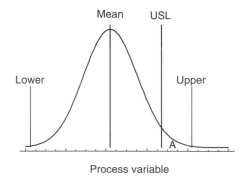

Process variable

Figure 9.2 Theoretical Gaussian distribution of a process variable. USL is the upper specification limit. A is the area of the curve to the right of USL that is equal to the probability of obtaining a value larger than USL. Lower is the mean minus 3 standard deviations, and Upper is the mean plus 3 standard deviations.

reasoning applies. The smaller the A, the better the quality of the process. By convention, this area is not measured directly. Instead, the ratio calculated as the specification limit's distance from the mean divided by three process standard deviations is used as a measure of the quality. For a USL we have

$$C_{pu} = \frac{USL - \mu}{3\sigma} \qquad (9.1)$$

and for an LSL we have

$$C_{pl} = \frac{\mu - LSL}{3\sigma} \qquad (9.2)$$

where C_{pu} and C_{pl} are called capability indices. It appears from Equation (9.1) and the definition of natural tolerance limits that $3\sigma = (USL - \mu)$ if C_{pu} is 1, implying that $(USL - \mu) = ('Upper' - \mu)$ or 'Upper' = USL, indicating 0.135 % of the values will be unacceptable. If the ratio is larger than one, less than 0.135 % will be unacceptable, and if it is less than one, more than 0.135 % will be unacceptable.

If a USL as well as an LSL are specified, the quality is assessed using C_{pk}, the smaller of the two values, C_{pu} and C_{pl}. Therefore, we have

$$C_{pk} = \min\{C_{pu}; C_{pl}\} \qquad (9.3)$$

Example 9.2

After revision of the treatment of the asthma patient from Example 2.7, the distribution of her PEFR values was stable, with a mean of 348.0 l/min and a standard deviation of 25.1 l/min. The LSL was 188.0 l/min. Therefore, the C_{pl} is $\frac{348.0 - 188.0}{3 \cdot 25.1} = 2.12$. If one assumes that the distribution is Gaussian and its parameters are known and not estimated as here, the standardised quantity (PEFR $-$ 348.0)/25.1 follows a Gaussian distribution with mean 0 and standard deviation 1. The standardised value of LSL is $\frac{188.0 - 348.0}{25.1} = -6.37$. Therefore, the probability of obtaining a value lower than 188.0 is $P(Z < -6.37)$, which is zero for all practical purposes. However, as indicated in Zhang et al. [5], the uncertainties of the capability index such as C_{pk} are relatively large and depend on the sample size. If possible, the capability indices should be calculated based on sample sizes of at least 50.

Example 9.3

In Example 3.2 the alignment of the femuro-tibial axis, following a total knee replacement (TKR) operation using robotic equipment, was followed in 78 patients. After a learning period, it appeared from the cumulative sum (CUSUM) curve that the process had stabilised. A CUSUM chart (not shown), using the remaining observations, demonstrated that the process was now in control, and an analysis of the distribution of the data showed that it did not deviate significantly from a Gaussian distribution. The mean and standard deviation of the data were 180.80° and 1.91°, respectively. If the specification limits are defined as $180.00° \pm 3.00° = [177.00°, 183.00°]$, we may calculate

$$C_{pu} = \frac{183.00 - 180.80}{3 \cdot 1.91} = 0.38$$

and

$$C_{pl} = \frac{180.80 - 177.00}{3 \cdot 1.91} = 0.66$$

Then $C_{pk} = \min\{0.38, 0.66\} = 0.38$. From an industrial point of view this is not a high quality process. However, in the healthcare sector one can't just delay the production until a suitable process has been developed, as long as the current treatment improves the patient's condition.

Example 9.4

In Example 1.2 the mean waiting time at an outpatient clinic was outside the control limits on Fridays. This problem was handled by reorganising and increasing the staffing of the outpatient clinic on Fridays. After this change had been made, the daily mean waiting times stabilised within the control limits with a mean of 15.72 min. and a standard deviation of 4.85 min. The government subsequently dictated a USL of 30 min. According to this standard, $C_{pu} = \frac{30.00 - 15.72}{3 \cdot 4.85} = 0.98$. This is a questionable level of quality according to industrial standards. However, as opposed to the above example, something can be done right away to improve the quality.

If the process variable is binary, the nominal value and tolerance limits may be related to p, the probability of the outcome, e.g., the death of the patient, and as long as the normal approximation applies the above equations may be used.

Example 9.5

Of 600 patients who received a liver transplant at a centre for transplantation, 90 died. We assume that the highest acceptable mortality rate is 0.20. This implies that USL $= 0.20$. $\hat{p}$ is $\frac{90}{600} = 0.15$.

The estimated standard deviation of $\hat{p}$ is

$$\sqrt{\frac{0.15 \cdot (1 - 0.15)}{600}} = 0.015$$

Therefore,

$$C_{pu} = \frac{0.20 - 0.15}{3 \cdot 0.015} = 1.14$$

According to industrial standards the quality is quite high, since the sample size is as large as 600.

9.2.2 Benchmarking Several Providers

If one collects data from several, say k, healthcare providers within the same organisation and measures the same process variable over time, one ends up with k samples.

Example 9.6

Table 9.1 shows, for a given period, the number of patients treated for AMI at each of 10 hospitals from the same health care organisation (column 2), the number discharged on aspirin as a secondary preventive

Table 9.1 Ten hospitals ranked according to appropriateness of treatment.

Number of patients discharged on aspirin (X)	Number of patients treated (n)	Rate of appropriate treatment	Rank of hospital
19	20	0.950	1
47	50	0.940	2
94	100	0.940	3
28	30	0.933	4
74	80	0.925	5
63	70	0.900	6
53	60	0.883	7
35	40	0.875	8
78	90	0.867	9
7	10	0.700	10
Sum (A): 498	Sum (B): 550	A/B: 0.906	

medication (column 1), and the fraction of patients receiving appropriate secondary aspirin medication (column 3). In column 4 the rank, according to rate of appropriate secondary preventive medication, is shown for each hospital. The data are invented.

Table 9.1 is an example of a league table. In commerce and sports, league tables have been used for many years to depict comparative performance. Recently, their use has also been extended to rank services provided by healthcare agencies. A league table may be defined as an established technique for displaying the comparative ranking of organisations in terms of their performance when standards against which to judge performance have not been set [6]. When assessing a given ranking, one should bear in mind that rank statistics have considerable inherent variability and sophisticated statistical methods (that are rarely used in practice) are needed to portray this variability [7, 8]. Therefore, rankings without this information are useless and may be extremely misleading. Adap *et al.* [6] pointed out that although the comparison of industrial products, e.g., different brands of automobiles, makes a lot of sense, this may not necessarily be true for healthcare products. The former are produced by systems that are basically different. The opposite is actually true for healthcare products. They argued that basically the systems used to produce the same type of healthcare product, e.g., surgical intervention in a specified type of patients, are (or should at least intend to be) similar because they are based on the same scientific evidence.

Assume that a given organisation of k healthcare providers behaves like a collection of k identical systems. Then, the principles described in the previous section may be applied. All samples from the k providers are first combined into one sample. Then the appropriate capability index is calculated using this sample. The necessary and sufficient conditions implied by the assumption are that the k processes corresponding to the k providers are all (1) in statistical control, and (2) all in the same state. The first condition may be tested, using a control chart for each provider. If each of the control charts depicts a process in statistical control, the first condition is fulfilled in all likelihood. Then, we need to assess if they are all in the same state. To do so, Adap *et al.* [6] suggested the use of control charts instead of the league tables. Continuing this line of thought, Spiegelhalter introduced the funnel plot for comparing institutional performance [9]. In this plot the observed sample statistic is plotted against a measure of its precision. Examples were given where proportions and changes in rates were compared [9]. The plot consists of a centreline equal to the overall average and 95 % and 99.8 % control limits relative to this centreline. They are calculated as a function of sample size, volume of cases, or population size depending on the application. It is assumed that all variation is random, i.e., only dependent on the average and the size of the sample, volume, or population. They form a funnel, demonstrating how the precision improves with volume. The observed provider values are finally plotted on this graph to produce the funnel plot. If all provider processes are in the same state of statistical control, the values ought to cluster at random relative to the centreline with approximately 5 % of the values being outside the 95 % limits and 0.2 % outside the 99.8 % limits.

Example 9.7

To construct an approximate funnel plot for the data from Table 9.1 we sorted them in ascending order according to sample size and depicted them on a p chart for variable sample size, with 99.8 % and 95 % control limits. The limits were calculated, using the normal approximation presented in Chapter 2.

Figure 9.3 shows the chart. One value (70 % with a sample size of 10) is below the lower 95 % limit, but within the 99.8 % limit. One out of 10 values between the 95 % and 99.8 % limits is not that unlikely if the process is in statistical control. Besides, the normal approximation does not hold in this example. The probability that X (the number of patients discharged on aspirin) is 7 or less out of a total of 10 is $1 - P(X > 7) = 1 - (P(X = 8) + P(X = 9) + P(X = 10)) = 0.0702$.

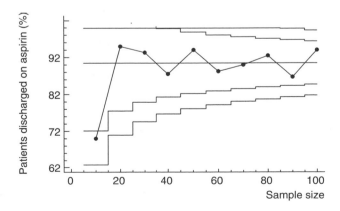

Figure 9.3 Percentage of acute myocardial infarction patients discharged on aspirin, depicted for each of 10 hospitals, on a p chart for variable sample size and 95 % (inner limits) and 99.8 % (outer limits) control limits.

So, in regard to secondary, preventive aspirin medication of AMI patients, the 10 hospitals are so well standardised that the between-hospital variation in outcome measure is purely random. Therefore, we may combine all samples into one, to obtain $\hat{p} = 0.906$ (see Table 9.1) with a standard deviation $= \sqrt{\frac{0.906 \cdot (1-0.906)}{550}} = 0.0124$. Then the quality of the organisation of hospitals may be assessed.

Example 9.8

The benchmark, i.e., the lowest acceptable percentage of AMI patients discharged on aspirin, was 85 % for the hospitals in the above example. Using Equation (9.2) on the values calculated in Example 9.7, we obtain $C_{pl} = \frac{0.906-0.850}{3 \cdot 0.0124} = 1.51$. Considering that the sample size is 550 this is an acceptable level of quality.

9.3 DEALING WITH PROCESSES THAT ARE NOT IN STATISTICAL CONTROL IN THE SAME STATE

The above example is the exception, rather than the rule.

Example 9.9

Figure 9.4(a) shows the percentage of AMI patients discharged on aspirin from each of 10 hospitals, depicted on a p chart for variable sample size. The benchmark is 85 %. The average is below this value. However, the hospitals are not in the same state of statistical control. If we remove samples # 4 and # 9, the values of which are outside the 99.8 % limits, and recalculate the control chart using the remaining data (chart not shown), the value of sample # 7 falls below the lower 99.8 % limit. Omitting sample # 7 and recalculating the control chart, we obtain the chart shown in Figure 9.4(b). Now the process is in control, at an acceptable high level. However, we need to find out why the three hospitals crossed the 99.8 % threshold.

It is imperative that the actions to be taken in response to a threshold being crossed are defined and written down as part of the design of a monitoring system. Otherwise even a well-designed system is very likely to be discredited through inappropriate use [10]. Prior to the construction of the funnel plot, the individual control chart of each

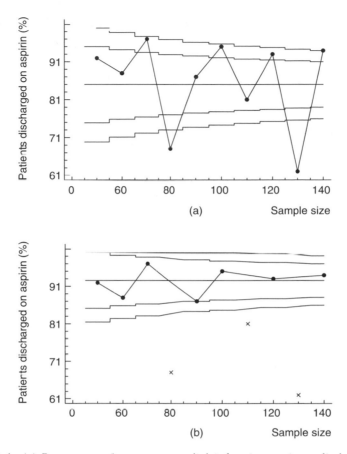

Figure 9.4 (a) Percentage of acute myocardial infarction patients discharged on aspirin, depicted for each of 10 hospitals on a *p* chart for variable sample size and 95 % (inner limits) and 99.8 % (outer limits) control limits. (b) Percentage of acute myocardial infarction patients discharged on aspirin, depicted for each of 7 hospitals on a *p* chart for variable sample size and 95 % (inner limits) and 99.8 % (outer limits) control limits. The crosses represent values that were outside the control limits of the original control chart (see Figure 9.4(a)) or the chart (not shown) calculated after the two outlying values of Figure 9.4(a) had been removed and the chart recalculated using the remaining 8 values. The control chart here was calculated without using these 3 values, which are depicted as crosses in the figure.

provider should be inspected to make sure that the process is in statistical control. If it is not, the cause of this should be investigated locally. Assuming that the funnel plot only includes data from processes that are in statistical control, a systematic search for special cause variation should be initiated for each outlying provider, i.e., it should be investigated why the process is in a state of statistical control that is different from that of the remaining providers.

In the example above we used a clinical process measure. This is a quality measure. Therefore, to assess the quality and search for the cause of outlying values is relatively straightforward. This is not so if a quality indicator like death rate or morbidity rate is used. In this case, crossing a threshold is not an indication of either high or low quality of care. No conclusions can be drawn until the reasons for the apparent deviation from the norm have been investigated. The first action to be taken, when searching for a special cause of variation, should always be to check the data carefully. Next, the case mix should be analysed. Then the structure and resources should be checked. For instance, one may calculate the number of physicians assigned per bed, etc. If a likely special cause has not yet been found, the actual process of care should be analyzed, and if this fails to give a result, it should be examined if individual healthcare persons could be the cause of the special variation [11]. However, as mentioned in the introduction, outcome measures like death rates and morbidity rates are poor proxies of quality of care, and to identify the cause of a deviating value may be difficult.

9.4 OVERDISPERSION

Figure 9.5, from a study by Spiegelhalter [12], shows the emergency readmission (within 30 days) rates following discharge from 140 National Health Service trusts from 2002 to 2003. To the left is shown a so-called forest plot showing 95 % confidence intervals, compared with the target overall average. To the right is shown the corresponding funnel plot, depicting percentage of readmitted versus number of discharges. The majority of institutions are located outside the control limits. The figure illustrates the phenomenon of overdispersion. The observed variation cannot be ascribed to random variation and a few outliers. This may typically be found when there is insufficient risk adjustment. Spiegelhalter suggests various possible ways of handling the situation [12]. An obvious solution is not to use the indicator. If this is not an option, one may try to improve the risk stratification by measuring risk factors that are contributing to the excess variation. Rather than comparing all institutions simultaneously, one may subdivide them into more homogeneous groups and produce a funnel plot for each group. This subdivision needs to be defined in advance in the protocol for the study and not deduced from the observed data. One might also define an interval of acceptable values and define outlying values as values lying outside this interval. This seems arbitrary and

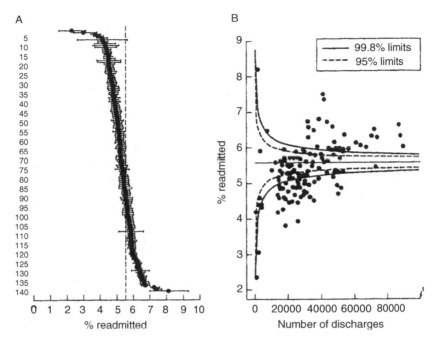

Figure 9.5 Emergency (within 30 days) readmission rates following discharge from 140 National Health Service acute trusts, 2002–2003. Reproduced with permission from Spiegelhalter DJ. Handling over-dispersion of performance indicators. Qual Saf Health Care 2005; 14:347–51.

does not take the sample sizes into consideration as the funnel plot does. The overdispersion may be estimated [13], so that the variation, assumed to be due to chance alone, is inflated to reflect the inevitable within-unit and between-units variation in outcome, due to unmeasured differences in case mix and other factors beyond the control of the unit. Ideally this should be estimated from historical data obtained from units, known to have had stable and acceptable performance levels. Alternatively, a technique may be used, whereby the effect on the estimate by outlying observations is somewhat dampened. The last approach is to assume that the institutions have their own true underlying rates, which are distributed around the overall average. The standard deviation of this distribution is estimated and used to adjust the control limits. The distribution may be estimated in various ways. One appealing approach might be to use a hierarchical model, as explained in Chapter 5. Clearly, statistical estimation of overdispersion is a temporary solution to be used when the causes of the excess variation are still being investigated.

9.5 MULTIPLE SIGNIFICANCE TESTING

In Chapter 1 and Chapter 3 we discussed the standard approach used to set alarm thresholds to optimise the trade-off between the in control average run length (ARL) and the ARL until a specified out-of-control condition is detected. Other approaches are also possible (see Frisen for a review [14]).

When several (k) units are monitored over time using a quality indicator such as the mortality rate, it is necessary to describe the expected rates of false alarms and successful detections among the k units being monitored. Marshall *et al.* [13] estimated the percentage of false alarms (*FDR* %) occurring by a given time, t, for CUSUM charts, and the percentage of out-of-control units that were successfully detected (*SDR* %). The threshold (h), the size of change (K) in terms of the number of process standard deviations the charts were designed to detect, and the percentage of units truly out of control (p_0) were all given. Tables showing *FDR* % and *SDR* % as a function of h, K, and p_0 would seem to be useful planning tools when designing an efficient monitoring system.

REFERENCES

[1] Kassirer JP. The use and abuse of practice profiles. N Engl J Med 1994; 330:634–6.
[2] James B. Information system concepts for quality measurement. Med Care 2003; 41(suppl):I-71–I-9.
[3] McGlynn EA. Selecting common measures of quality and system performance. Med Care 2002; 41(suppl):I-39–I-47.
[4] Christiansen CL, and Morris CN. Improving the statistical approach to health care provider profiling. Ann Intern Med 1997; 127:764–8.
[5] Zhang NF, Stenback GA, and Wardrop DM. Interval estimation of process capability index Cpk. Commun Stat Meth 1990; 19:4455–70.
[6] Adap P, Rouse AM, Mohammed MA, and Marshall T. Performance league tables: the NHS deserves better. BMJ 2002; 324:95–8.
[7] Goldstein H, and Spiegelhalter DJ. League tables and their limitations: statistical issues in comparisons of institutional performance J Roy Stat Soc A 1996; 159:385–443.
[8] Marshall EC, and Spiegelhalter DJ. Reliability of league tables of in vitro fertilisation clinics: retrospective analysis of live birth rates. BMJ 1998; 316:1701–5.
[9] Spiegelhalter D. Funnel plots for comparing institutional performance. Stat Med 2005; 24:1185–202.
[10] Spiegelhalter DJ. Monitoring clinical performance: a commentary. J Thorac Cardiovasc Surg 2004; 128:820–2.

[11] Lilford R, Mohammed MA, Spiegelhalter DJ, and Thomsen R. Use and misuse of process and outcome data in managing performance of acute medical care: avoiding institutional stigma. Lancet 2004; 363:1147–54.

[12] Spiegelhalter DJ. Handling over-dispersion of performance indicators. Qual Saf Health Care 2005; 14:347–51.

[13] Marshall EC, Best N, Bottle A, and Aylin P. Statistical issues in the monitoring of health outcomes across multiple units. J Roy Stat Soc A 2004; 167:541–59.

[14] Frisen M. Evaluations of methods for statistical surveillance. Stat Med 1992; 11:1489–502.

Appendix A – Basic Statistical Concepts

Test sampling is a central theme in statistical quality improvement. Test samples are selected to provide information about the population from which they are taken. A test sample may be used to characterise the population and test a hypothesis about its characteristics. In the present context, we are interested in the population of products produced by some process. The process is considered a mechanism, which produces products in a random way, meaning that each single product deviates more or less from a product that is typical for the process and the deviations appear at random and independent of each other.

Statements about a process based on a single test sample are encumbered with uncertainty. Therefore, it is necessary to employ statistical methods to describe and quantify this uncertainty. The purpose of this chapter is to familiarise the reader with these methods and enable him/her to understand their application. We introduce the basic statistical concepts using an example.

A.1 AN EXAMPLE OF RANDOM SAMPLING

Assume that we want to buy a shipment of 5000 disposable electrodes, for the measurement of electrocardiograms (ECG). An electrode is defective if it cannot transmit the voltage to the meter. Before we decide

Statistical Development of Quality in Medicine   P. Winkel and N. F. Zhang
© 2007 John Wiley & Sons, Ltd

whether or not to buy the shipment, we want to be reasonably sure that the percentage of defective electrodes is sufficiently low. Once an electrode is tested, it becomes destructed and cannot be used again. Therefore, a complete inspection of the shipment implies that tested electrodes are destructed. How do we get reliable information about the shipment, without destroying all the electrodes?

A natural approach would be to select a test sample of electrodes and calculate the percentage of defective electrodes in the sample. In order to obtain a representative test sample, it has to be selected at random. Selected at random means that all possible equally sized test samples have the same probability of being selected. Based on the available information, the percentage of defective electrodes found in the test sample is our best guess of the unknown percentage of the shipment. It is referred to as an estimate of the true, but unknown percentage.

How uncertain is this estimate? The uncertainty depends on the size of the test sample. Intuitively this makes sense. The following simplistic reasoning does not prove the contention, but it supports the intuition. The larger the test sample is, the more possibilities are covered, and the larger is the chance of getting close to the truth. If the test sample comprises one electrode, the possibilities covered include 0 or 1 defective electrode, or 0 % and 100 %, respectively. If it comprises 10 electrodes, the possibilities include 0 %, 10 %, 20 %, etc. up to and including 100 % defective electrodes in the test sample, etc.

Using statistical reasoning, one may calculate an interval around the percentage found that covers the true percentage with an a priori specified high probability, e.g., 99 %. This interval is referred to as a confidence interval. The larger the sample is, the narrower this interval will be. Assume one is content if the percentage of defective electrodes is not larger than 3 %. If a confidence interval is 0 % to 2 %, and the probability that the true value is included in the interval is 99.9 %, we will, of course, accept the shipment.

Assume that we want to assess the hypothesis that the percentage of defective electrodes in the above shipment is 3 %, and we have available a test sample with five electrodes. There are six possible compositions of a sample of five; it may comprise 0, 1, 2, 3, 4, or 5 defective electrodes. Zero is the most likely result if the hypothesis is true; it is closest to 3 %. Then follows 1 (20 % of the test sample), 2 (40 %), 3 (60 %), 4 (80 %), and 5 (100 %). The probability that we will obtain a sample of a given composition may be calculated under the assumption that our hypothesis is true. Doing so for this example, we obtain a distribution of six probabilities.

When testing the hypothesis we apply this probability distribution. We calculate the probability that we will obtain a sample of the same composition as our sample or one that is more extreme (i.e., with more defectives). If this probability is very small, we reject the hypothesis. For example, if the hypothesis is true, the probability of getting a sample containing two or more defective electrodes is less than 1 %. Therefore, in this case we reject the hypothesis. The weakness of this approach is obvious. For example, the probability that we will obtain a sample comprising two or more defective electrodes will still be very small (8.15 %), even if the true percentage is as high as 10 %. Conversely, the probability of accepting the hypothesis is about 92 %. Therefore, in this example there is a high probability of erroneously accepting the hypothesis, unless the actual percentage deviates considerably from the hypothesised one. One says that the power of the test is weak.

A.2   DATA

A sample of products may be characterised by classifying each one into one of several possible categories, e.g., defective versus nondefective products, or by measuring one or more significant properties. The result is a set of data, comprising numerically coded properties and/or the values of measurements. It may be expedient to inspect the data and calculate various quantities, summarising important properties of the dataset.

A.2.1   Extreme Values (Outliers)

Prior to the description of a dataset, it may be appropriate to inspect it for outliers. An outlier in a set of data is defined as an observation (or subset of observations), which appears to be inconsistent with the remainder of that set of data [1]. Outliers may be identified using a dot diagram. A dot diagram consists of an abscissa on which the values are depicted as dots.

Outliers may arise due to errors (analytical errors, clerical errors, miscalculations, etc.) or because of the out-of-the-ordinary patterns of the probability distributions.

In the first case, the error should be corrected if it is possible. Otherwise the result should be discarded. For example, a relatively inexperienced person may commit an error. In the second case, the outliers are related to the distribution that the observations are assumed to follow, e.g., the normal distribution. When deciding whether an outlier should be discarded or not, the sensible approach is to identify the reason why the observation is an outlier. If this is not possible, one may test the hypothesis that a value as extreme as the one observed belongs to the same category of values as the remaining ones. Several tests of discordance are available, e.g., Dixon's test [1]. If a plausible explanation cannot be found, one should be very cautious in discarding a measurement. But of course, it may be obvious that the measurement is wrong. If the weight of a 30-year-old man has been recorded as 0.65 kilo, e.g., one may reject this outlier.

A.2.2 The Distribution of Data

When the dataset has been scanned for outliers and those (if any) found have been dealt with one way or the other, the distribution of the data should be examined. To illustrate how this may be done, we will use a dataset lent to us by Steen Watt-Boolsen (Department of Surgery at Nykøbing Falster Central Hospital, Denmark). The data include the results of various clinical observations made in 870 consecutive surgical patients. The state of each patient prior to operation has been characterised by a physiological score, which is a function of laboratory measurements and clinical signs, and each operation has been characterised, using a scoring system that quantifies its extent and severity [2].

Table A.1 shows how the distribution of the physiological scores has been characterised. The measurements have been sorted according to size and classified into a suitable number of intervals. The table shows the intervals (upper and lower limits and centre values) and the number of observations classified into each interval (frequencies), i.e., the frequency distribution.

Figure A.1 depicts a histogram showing the frequency distribution of the physiological scores of the above-mentioned 870 patients. The horizontal axis of real numbers is divided into a number of intervals. A histogram depicts the number of observations (the frequency) included in each of these intervals as vertical bars in a co-ordinate system. The x-axis represents the values and the ordinate the frequencies. A histogram captures the shape of the distribution of the data, its location, and its spread. A simple rule to apply, when choosing the number of intervals, is to use the integer closest to the square root of the number of observations. It is also appropriate to use equally sized intervals and let the first one begin slightly to the left to the smallest of the observations. If the number

Table A.1 Tabular representation of the values of the physiological score measured in 870 surgical patients.

Interval				Distributions			
Number [i]	Lower limit	Upper limit	Middle point	Frequency [x_i]	Relative frequency [$\frac{x_i}{n}$]	Cumulative frequency [Σx_i]	Cumulative relative frequency [$\Sigma \frac{x_i}{n}$]
1	10.0	12.0	11.0	47	0.0540	47	0.0540
2	12.0	14.0	13.0	150	0.1724	197	0.2264
3	14.0	16.0	15.0	134	0.1540	331	0.3805
4	16.0	18.0	17.0	98	0.1126	429	0.4931
5	18.0	20.0	19.0	61	0.0701	490	0.5632
6	20.0	22.0	21.0	63	0.0724	553	0.6356
7	22.0	24.0	23.0	58	0.0667	611	0.7023
8	24.0	26.0	25.0	64	0.0736	675	0.7759
9	26.0	28.0	27.0	49	0.0563	724	0.8322
10	28.0	30.0	29.0	35	0.0402	759	0.8724
11	30.0	32.0	31.0	33	0.0379	792	0.9103
12	32.0	34.0	33.0	24	0.0276	816	0.9379
13	34.0	36.0	35.0	14	0.0161	830	0.9540
14	36.0	38.0	37.0	9	0.0103	839	0.9644
15	38.0	40.0	39.0	7	0.0080	846	0.9724
16	40.0	42.0	41.0	5	0.0057	851	0.9782
17	42.0	44.0	43.0	7	0.0080	858	0.9862
18	44.0	46.0	45.0	6	0.0069	864	0.9931
19	46.0	48.0	47.0	3	0.0034	867	0.9966
20	48.0	50.0	49.0	0	0.0000	867	0.9966
21	50.0	52.0	51.0	1	0.0011	868	0.9977
22	52.0	54.0	53.0	0	0.0000	868	0.9977
23	54.0	56.0	55.0	1	0.0011	869	0.9989
24	56.0	58.0	57.0	0	0.0011	870	1.0000

x_i is the number of observations, i.e., the frequency of the ith interval. n is the number of observations. $\frac{x_i}{n}$ is the relative frequency of the ith interval, $\sum_{j=1}^{i} x_j$ is the ith cumulative frequency, i.e., the number of observations smaller than or equal to the upper limit of the ith interval, and $\sum_{j=1}^{i} \frac{x_j}{n}$ is the ith cumulative relative frequency.

of intervals is too small, one may lose information. On the other hand, if it is too large, important features may be hidden by unimportant details.

Example A.1

The following dataset includes 9 values that have been ordered according to size

$$\{1, 3, 5, 5, 6, 7, 9, 10, 11\}.$$

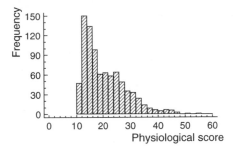

Figure A.1 The frequency distribution of 870 physiological scores.

We want to calculate the frequency distribution, the relative frequency distribution, the cumulative distribution, and the relative cumulative distribution (see Table A.1 for definitions). We classify the observations into three ($\sqrt{9}$) equally sized intervals

$$0 \leq x < 4, 4 \leq x < 8, \text{and } 8 \leq x < 12.$$

The first two values belong to the first interval, the following four to the second interval, and the last three to the third interval. Therefore, the three frequencies are:
2, 4, and 3, and the corresponding relative frequencies are

$$\frac{2}{9}, \frac{4}{9}, \text{ and } \frac{3}{9}.$$

The cumulative frequencies are calculated by counting the number of values in each of the following intervals

$$0 \leq x < 4, 0 \leq x < 8, \text{and } 0 \leq x < 12.$$

Two values are less than 4, $(2 + 4)$ are less than 8, and $(2 + 4 + 3)$ less than 12. Therefore, the three cumulative frequencies are: 2, 6, and 9. The corresponding cumulative, relative frequencies are

$$\frac{2}{9}, \frac{2+4}{9}, \text{ and } \frac{2+4+3}{9}.$$

A.2.3 The Location of the Data

Various quantities may be used to summarise the location of a set of measurement values. The most commonly used ones are the mean, the median, and the mode. The mean is the centre of gravity of the frequency distribution. It is calculated as the arithmetic average ($\bar{x}$) of the measurements, using the equation

$$\bar{x} = \sum_{i=1}^{n} \frac{x_i}{n} \tag{A.1}$$

where x_i is the ith measurement and n the number of measurements. The median is the middle value in the ordered sequence of the data if the number of observations is an odd number and it is the arithmetic mean of the two middle values if it is an even number. The mode is the most frequently occurring value (or set of values) in the data material.

Example A.2

The mean value of the data set {1, 2, 3, 3, 3, 4, 4, 5, 6, 7} is

$$\frac{1 + 2 + 3 + 3 + 3 + 4 + 4 + 5 + 6 + 7}{10} = 3.8.$$

The median is

$$\frac{3 + 4}{2} = 3.5.$$

The mode is 3.

A.2.4 The Spread of Data

The spread of measurement values is often characterised using the range, the variance, or the standard deviation. The range is defined as the difference between the largest and the smallest value in the data set. This quantity only depends on two of the measurement values. If there are more than two measurement values in a set of data, information will be lost if we only use two of them.

Another approach, utilising all data points, is to calculate the square of the distance between the result of each measurement and the mean value, add the squares, and divide their sum by $(n - 1)$ where n is the number of squares. The result is denoted by s^2 and called the variance. To obtain the same unit as that of the measurements, the standard deviation (s) may be calculated as

$$s = \sqrt{\frac{\sum_{i=1}^{n} (x_i - \bar{x})^2}{n - 1}} \qquad \text{(A.2)}$$

The standard deviation is a measure of the location of the values relative to the mean value. Since it is more convenient to use a quantity having the same unit as the results of the measurements, the standard deviation is usually the quantity of choice.

The quantity $(n - 1)$ is sometimes referred to as the degrees of freedom (df) when the distribution of the data is normal (see A.3.4.1). The df expresses the amount of information available in the sample.

Example A.3

The set of data $\{1, 3, 4, 8\}$ has a range equal to $8 - 1 = 7$. To calculate the variance, we first calculate the mean

$$\bar{x} = \frac{1 + 3 + 4 + 8}{4} = 4.$$

The sum of the squares is: $(1 - 4)^2 + (3 - 4)^2 + (4 - 4)^2 + (8 - 4)^2 = 26$. Since $n = 4$, we have

$$s^2 = \frac{26}{4 - 1} = 8.67 \text{ and } s = \sqrt{8.67} = 2.94.$$

A.3 PROBABILITY DISTRIBUTIONS

As we saw in the introductory example, it may be of interest to calculate the probability of obtaining specified values when a sample is selected at random from a population and the value of some quantity is measured in each item of the sample.

Example A.4

A municipality includes 50 000 inhabitants above the age of 16 years. It is known that their body weights are distributed as follows (see Table A.2):

Table A.2 Weight/kg of 50 000 municipality inhabitants above the age of 16 years.

Interval	Frequency	Probability (relative frequency)	Cumulative frequency	Cumulative probability (cumulative relative frequency)
50 – 70	5000	0.10	5.000	0.10
71 – 80	15 000	0.30	20.000	0.40
81 – 90	20 000	0.40	40.000	0.80
91 – 100	6000	0.12	46.000	0.92
101 – 130	4000	0.08	50.000	1.00

Mean value 83.2 kg. Standard deviation 11.5 kg.

5000 are between 50 kg and 70 kg, 15 000 between 71 and 80 kg, 20 000 between 81 and 90 kg, 6000 between 91 and 100 kg, and 4000 between 100 and 130 kg. The identity of each person and the corresponding weight has been stored in a database. Using this database, we select one of the 50 000 persons so that each person has the same probability of being selected. What is the probability that the person's weight is between 71 and 80 kg?

All inhabitants have the same chance of being selected, and 15 000 out of the 50 000 weigh between 71 and 80 kg. Therefore, the probability is $\frac{15\,000}{50\,000} = 0.3$. Using the same type of reasoning, one may calculate the probability that an inhabitant weighs between 50 and 70 kg as: $\frac{5000}{50\,000} = 0.1$, that he/she weighs between 81 and 90 kg as: $\frac{20\,000}{50\,000} = 0.4$, etc.

Table A.2 has been constructed using the above database and the same principles as in Table A.1. The difference between the two tables is that Table A.1 shows the distribution of a random sample, whereas Table A.2 shows the distribution of a whole population. Therefore, the latter is a probability distribution. A probability in Table A.2 corresponds to the relative frequency in Table A.1, and a cumulative probability corresponds to the cumulative relative frequency. A cumulative probability is defined as the probability of selecting an inhabitant whose weight is equal to or less than the upper weight limit of the category (see column 1, Table A.2). For instance, the probability of selecting an inhabitant whose weight is equal to or less than 90 kg may be read from the table. It is 0.8.

In the above, we defined a mathematical model comprising a distribution of probabilities and of cumulative probabilities that may be used to calculate the probabilities of obtaining various outcomes when sampling from the population. The weight of each individual is stored in the database. Therefore, we may want to better utilise the available information.

If we use the rule of thumb for constructing a histogram, we need to have $\sqrt{50\,000}$ equally sized intervals, i.e., about 224. The range of the weights is $130 - 50 = 80$ kg. Therefore, the interval size should be $\frac{80}{224} = 0.36$ kg for the intervals to cover the values of interest. The first interval should begin slightly to the left of the smallest value, 50 kg.

Example A.5

An urn contains 3000 red and 5000 white balls, i.e., a total of 8000 balls. A ball is selected from the urn so that all balls have the same probability of being selected, and its colour is noted. What is the probability that it is red? Since 3000 of the 8000 balls are red and all balls have the same probability of being selected, the probability is: $\frac{3000}{8000} = 0.375$. Imagine that the ratio of red and white balls is not known and we want to obtain an educated guess of the probability of selecting a red ball. To do so, we use a mathematical model, stating that the probability of selecting a red ball is p $(0 < p < 1)$.

To get information about p, we conduct 50 independent experiments. Each experiment consists of picking a ball at random from the urn, noting its colour, replacing the ball, and mixing all balls thoroughly. It turns out that 21 of the 50 balls are red. Therefore, we guess that p, the fraction of red balls in the urn, is as demonstrated experimentally, i.e., $\frac{21}{50} = 0.420$. The relative deviation between our estimate and the truth is: $\frac{0.420-0.375}{0.375} = 12\,\%$. Our estimate is encumbered by uncertainty.

A sample selected as described above is referred to as a random sample with replacement. As shown in the above examples, a probability distribution is a mathematical model of the relation between the result of an observation and the probability that we will obtain this value when a random sample is selected from a specified population. This may be expressed in a more formal way. We define a random variable, X. This variable takes on a value each time we conduct our experiment. In Example A.4, the value was equal to the weight of the subject selected, and in Example A.5 it was equal to the number of red balls in the sample. The probability distribution is used to calculate the probability that the random variable will take on a specified value or some value within a

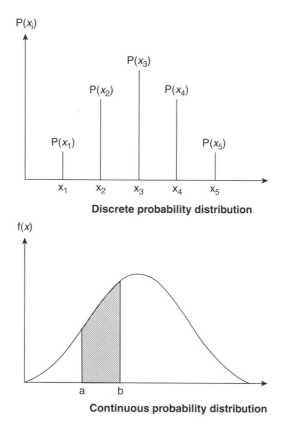

Figure A.2   A discrete (upper frame) and a continuous (lower frame) probability distribution.

specified interval of values. If the number of possible values is either finite or infinite but countable, the corresponding distribution is referred to as a discrete probability distribution, and otherwise it is referred to as a continuous probability distribution.

Figure A.2 depicts a discrete (upper frame) and a continuous (lower frame) probability distribution. Each of the possible values in a discrete distribution is associated with a probability $(P(X = x_i))$, i.e., the probability that the random variable (X) will take on this particular value. The sum of all the probabilities is 1, because it is certain that X will take on one of the possible values. A continuous distribution is depicted as a continuous curve in a co-ordinate system where the ordinate depicts the probability density function $f(x)$ and the abscissa, the values that X may take on. The area under the curve is 1 (the probability that X will take on one of the possible values). The probability that the random variable will take on a value within a specified interval (e.g., the interval from a to b with $a < b$ in Figure A.2) is calculated by measuring the corresponding area under the curve, i.e., the probability

$$P(a \leq X \leq b) = \int_a^b f(x)dx \qquad (A.3)$$

There are many different types of probability distributions. A random sample provides information about the type that may best characterise the population from which the sample was obtained. The shape of the histogram of the data will resemble that of the proper probability distribution. The larger the sample, the better the resemblance tends to be. This fact may be utilised in practice because inspection of the histogram of the sample data may reveal which type of probability distribution could be useful to apply.

Example A.6

A random variable may take on one of the values, 1, 2, 3, 4, and 5. The corresponding probability distribution includes the probabilities

$$P(X = 1) = 0.1, P(X = 2) = 0.4, P(X = 3) = 0.3, P(X = 4) = 0.1,$$

and

$$P(X = 5) = 0.1.$$

What are the values of $P(X = 7)$, $P(X < 3)$, and $P(2 < X \leq 4)$?

Seven does not belong to the values that X may assume. Therefore, $P(X = 7) = 0$. The values smaller than 3, that X may assume, are 1 and 2. Hence, we have,

$$P(X < 3) = P(X = 1) + P(X = 2) = 0.1 + 0.4 = 0.5.$$

Using a similar line of reasoning, we find that

$$P(2 < X \leq 4) = P(X = 3) + P(X = 4) = 0.3 + 0.1 = 0.4.$$

A.3.1 The Mean Value and Standard Deviation of a Probability Distribution

Just as we characterised the location of a data set by calculating its mean value, we may characterise the location of a probability distribution by calculating its mean value.

The mean value of a probability distribution is defined as its centre of gravity. If the distribution is discrete, the mean is defined by the equation

$$\mu = \sum_{i=1}^{k} P(x_i)x_i \qquad (A.4)$$

where k is the number of discrete probabilities of the distribution. If the distribution is continuous, the mean is defined by

$$\mu = \int_{a}^{b} xf(x)dx \qquad (A.5)$$

where a and b are the lower and upper limits of the random variable X.

A measure of the spread of a distribution is its variance, σ^2. The variance of a discrete distribution is defined by

$$\sigma^2 = \sum_{i=1}^{k} P(x_i)(x_i - \mu)^2 \qquad (A.6)$$

The variance of a continuous distribution is defined by

$$\sigma^2 = \int_{a}^{b} f(x)(x - \mu)^2 dx \qquad (A.7)$$

The standard deviation of a probability distribution is defined by

$$\sigma = \sqrt{\sigma^2} \qquad (A.8)$$

A.3.2 Parameters

A specified type of mathematical function, e.g., a linear one, may be defined using a formula that includes one or more parameters. A linear function which is graphically represented by a line, is defined by the formula $y = a + bx$, where a and b are the parameters of the function. A linear function is uniquely defined by specifying the values that the parameters should assume. If we define $a = 2$ and $b = 3$, we have specified the linear function $y = 2 + 3x$. Therefore, we have a 'family' of functions where each member is uniquely defined by the values assumed by the parameters. In the same way, a specified type of probability distribution may be defined as a family of probability distributions where each distribution is uniquely defined by the values assumed by the parameters.

Example A.7

A random variable (X) may assume the values 1 and 0. The corresponding family of probability distributions is defined by the formulas

$$P(X = 1) = p \text{ and } P(X = 0) = (1 - p) \text{ (for } 0 < p < 1)$$

where p is the parameter of the distributions. For each value that p may
assume, a corresponding probability distribution exists. If $p = 0.4$, the
corresponding   discrete   distribution   includes   the   probabilities
$P(X = 1) = 0.4$ and $P(X = 0) = 0.6$.

In many situations, there are good reasons to believe that one's data
are generated by a mechanism that may be approximated by a given type
of probability distribution, e.g., the Gaussian one (see Section A.3.4.1).
However, the parameter values, characterising the distribution, are not
known. Using a randomly selected sample from the population, one may
calculate an estimate of each parameter from the sample values so that
each estimate is the best guess of the true value of the parameter, given
the available information. The function used is referred to as an estimator. It is crucial for the reliability of the conclusions, drawn on the basis
of a sample, that it is truly a random one (i.e., randomly selected).
     A sample is a random sample if each value is produced independently of
all other values, and all values are generated by the same probability
distribution. This is true if the population, from which the sample is taken,
is infinite. If the population is finite (e.g., an urn of balls), each element in
the sample should be replaced before the next one is selected (see Example
A.5). If a sample is taken without replacement, all possible samples of the
same size should have the same probability of being selected.
     An estimator is in itself a random variable. Therefore, the possible values
that it may assume may be characterised by a probability distribution. An
unbiased estimator follows a probability distribution with a mean value
(see Section A.3.2) which is the true value of the parameter. Among all
possible unbiased estimators, the best one is the one with the probability
distribution that has the smallest standard deviation (see Section A.3.2).
     We will present some important families of probability distributions
that are often applied in statistical quality improvement. In each case, we
explain when to apply the type of distribution and how its parameters
may be estimated using a random sample from the population.

A.3.3 Examples of Discrete Distributions

The most commonly used discrete distributions in quality control and
assurance are the binomial distribution and the Poisson distribution.

A.3.3.1   The binomial distribution

Application Assume that a sample comprising n products is selected from a product line. Each product is classified as defective or nondefective. Here, it would be natural to use the binomial distribution when analysing the data.

Probabilities, parameter, mean value, and standard deviation Consider an experiment that has two possible outcomes. The probability of one outcome is p ($0 < p < 1$) and that of the other outcome is $(1 - p)$. The experiment may include tossing of a coin and noting if the result is head or tail. Another example could be a surgical procedure where it is noted if the patient survives or not. To characterise the experiment, we define a random variable Y that may assume one of two possible values, 0 or 1. Y follows a discrete probability distribution where $P(Y = 1)$ is p and $P(Y = 0)$ is $1 - p$. We now define a slightly more complicated experiment, comprising a specified number (n) of independent repetitions of the above-mentioned type of experiment. The same two-point discrete probability distribution characterises each experiment.

To describe the possible outcomes of the sequence of n independent experiments, we define a new random variable X. The value of X is equal to the number of experiments that have the same specified outcome, e.g., that the patient died, or the result was head when we tossed a coin. The possible values that X may assume include the values 0, 1, 2, etc., up to and including n. The probability distribution of X is discrete, and it includes $n + 1$ discrete probabilities. It is referred to as the binomial distribution. The probability distribution in Section A.1 is an example of a binomial distribution with parameters $n = 5$ and $p = 0.03$. To calculate the probability that X attains some value x, we first calculate the number of different combinations that may be obtained where x experiments give the specified outcome and the remaining $n - x$ experiments do not. This may be calculated using the formula

$$\binom{n}{x} = \frac{n!}{x!(n - x)!}$$

where $n! = 1 \cdot 2 \cdot \cdots \cdot (n - 1)n$. $0! = 1$. The probability of each of these combinations is calculated using the equation

$$p^x(1 - p)^{n-x} \tag{A.9}$$

Hence, the probability that $X = x$ is the product between the number of different combinations and the probability given in Expression (A.9). We have

$$P(X = x) = \frac{n!}{x!(n-x)!} p^x (1-p)^{n-x} \qquad (A.10)$$

It may be shown that the mean value of the binomial distribution is

$$\mu - np \qquad (A.11)$$

and that the standard deviation is

$$\sigma = \sqrt{np(1-p)} \qquad (A.12)$$

Example A.8

X is a random variable following a binomial distribution with $p = 0.1$ and $n = 5$. We want to calculate the probability $P(X \leq 1)$. We have $P(X \leq 1) = P(X = 0) + P(X = 1)$ where each of these probabilities may be computed, using Equation (A.10). Adding the results, we obtain the probability requested

$$P(X \leq 1) = \sum_{k=0}^{1} \frac{5!}{k!(5-k)!} 0.1^k 0.9^{5-k}$$

$$= \frac{5!}{0!5!} 0.1^0 0.9^5 + \frac{5!}{1!4!} 0.1^1 0.9^4$$

$$= 0.59049 + 0.32805 = 0.91854.$$

Sometimes, it may be more meaningful to report the fraction of defective products $\left(\frac{X}{n}\right)$ in place of X, the number of defective products. If the random variable X follows a binomial distribution with parameters p and n, the distribution of $\frac{X}{n}$ may be derived, and it may be shown that this distribution has the mean value p and standard deviation equal to $\sqrt{\frac{p(1-p)}{n}}$.

Estimates The parameters of the binomial distribution are n and p. The estimator of p

$$\hat{p} = \frac{X}{n} \qquad (A.13)$$

X is the number of experiments that had the specified outcome. Inserting the value of this estimate in Equations (A.11) and (A.12), estimates of the mean and the standard deviation may be obtained, respectively.

A.3.3.2 The Poisson distribution

Applications The Poisson distribution is often applicable in situations where one examines the number of times a random phenomenon is occurring per unit, e.g., the number of disintegrations of a radioactive substance per time unit, the number of colonies of bacteria per unit of volume, the number of patients admitted to a department per time unit, etc.

Probabilities, parameter, mean value, and standard deviation We define a random variable (X) equal to the number of times the random phenomenon is observed per unit. Assuming that X follows a Poisson distribution, it may be shown that the probability that X attains a given value, x, may be calculated using the equation

$$P(X = x) = \frac{e^{-\lambda}\lambda^x}{x!} \tag{A.14}$$

where λ ($\lambda > 0$) is the parameter of the Poisson distribution. The probability that X will assume a value equal to or less than a specified positive integer k is calculated as

$$P(X \le k) = \sum_{x=0}^{k} \frac{e^{-\lambda}\lambda^x}{x!} \tag{A.15}$$

It may be shown that the mean value of a Poisson distribution (μ) is equal to λ and the standard deviation (σ) is equal to $\sqrt{\lambda}$. We have

$$\mu = \lambda \tag{A.16}$$

and

$$\sigma = \sqrt{\lambda} \tag{A.17}$$

Estimates The parameter λ is estimated using the equation

$$\hat{\lambda} = \sum_{i=1}^{n} \frac{X_i}{n} \tag{A.18}$$

where X_I is the number of times the random phenomenon was observed in the ith unit, and n is the number of units examined. The standard deviation is estimated, by replacing λ by $\hat{\lambda}$ in Equation (A.17).

Example A.9

Assume we want to follow the number of medical complications that occur during and immediately after a surgical procedure and we choose 15 consecutive surgical patients as our inspection unit.

The number of medical complications occurring per unit of patients is assumed to follow a Poisson distribution. Table A.3 shows the number of medical complications in each of 20 consecutive inspection units. Using Equation (A.18) we may obtain an estimate of the mean of the Poisson distribution, and inserting the result in Equation (A.17) we may obtain an estimate of the standard deviation. The sum of complications observed in the 20 inspection units is 129. Therefore, λ is estimated as $\frac{129}{20} = 6.50$ medical complication/unit. The standard deviation is $\sqrt{6.5} = 2.55$ medical complication/unit.

Table A.3 The number of medical complications occurring in each of 20 patient groups.

Patient group #	Number of medical complications
1	4
2	4
3	5
4	9
5	10
6	8
7	7
8	6
9	2
10	7
11	9
12	8
13	7
14	7
15	6
16	7
17	3
18	5
19	13
20	3
Sum	129

A.3.4　Examples of Continuous Distributions

The Gaussian or normal distribution is by far the most widely used distribution in quality control and assurance.

A.3.4.1　The Gaussian (normal) distribution

Applications The result of the measurement of a given quantity may be expected to follow a Gaussian distribution if the measurement procedure is jointly influenced by many independent factors, none of which domineers the remaining ones.

Probabilities, parameters, mean value, and standard deviation A Gaussian distribution is characterised by two parameters, μ and σ. It is defined by the following equation

$$\int_{-\infty}^{\infty} f(x)dx = \int_{-\infty}^{\infty} \frac{1}{\sqrt{2\pi}\sigma} e^{\frac{(x-\mu)^2}{2\sigma^2}} dx = 1 \qquad (A.19)$$

where $f(x)$ is the probability density function. Graphically the distribution is depicted as a bell shaped, symmetrical curve (see Figure A.3).

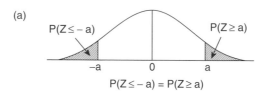

(a)

$P(Z \le -a)$　　　　　　　　$P(Z \ge a)$

$-a$　　　0　　　a

$P(Z \le -a) = P(Z \ge a)$

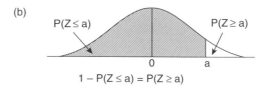

(b)

$P(Z \le a)$　　　　　　　　$P(Z \ge a)$

0　　　a

$1 - P(Z \le a) = P(Z \ge a)$

Figure A.3　Graphical illustration of two rules used to calculate probabilities of a random variable (Z) following a standardised Gaussian distribution with mean 0 and standard deviation 1.

It may be shown that the centre of gravity of the distribution, i.e., the mean value, is μ and that the standard deviation is σ. It may also be shown that 68.26 % of the area of the distribution is located within the interval $\mu \pm \sigma$, 95.46 % of the area within the interval $\mu \pm 2\sigma$, and 99.73 % within the interval $\mu \pm 3\sigma$.

To calculate the probability of obtaining a value within a specified interval [a, b], one needs to calculate the corresponding area of the distribution, i.e., to integrate $f(x)$ from a to b. To do so, it is necessary first to transform the original random variable X. The transformed variable, Z is given by the equation

$$Z = \frac{X - \mu}{\sigma} \tag{A.20}$$

Because the original interval is [a, b], the density function of the transformed variable Z, must be integrated from $\frac{a-\mu}{\sigma}$ to $\frac{b-\mu}{\sigma}$ to obtain the desired probability. It may be shown that Z follows a Gaussian distribution with mean 0 and standard deviation 1 (the standardised Gaussian distribution). The probability that Z assumes a value equal to or less than a specified value (z) is calculated by integrating the distribution from $-\infty$ to z. This probability is shown in Table A.4 for various values of Z.

The probability distribution is symmetrical around zero. Therefore, we have, $p(Z \leq -a) = p(Z \geq a)$ (see Figure A.3 (a)). Furthermore: $p(Z \geq a) = 1 - p(Z \leq a)$ (see Figure A.3 (b)). The correctness of these rules is directly apparent from Figure A.3.

Example A.10

It is known that $P(Z \leq 3) = 0.99865$. We want to find the value of $P(Z \leq -3)$. According to Figure A.3 we have $P(Z \leq -3) = P(Z \geq 3)$ and according to the same figure, $P(Z \geq 3) = 1 - P(Z \leq 3)$. The desired probability is: $1 - 0.99865 = 0.00135$. We have

$$P(Z \geq 3) = p(Z \leq -3) = 0.00135$$

Example A.11

A random variable X follows a Gaussian distribution with mean 10 and standard deviation 2. We want to calculate the probability that X

Table A.4 The cumulative distribution $(\Phi(Z) = P(Z \leq z))$ of the Gaussian distribution with mean $= 0$ and standard deviation $= 1$.

	$100\Phi(Z)$									
z	0.00	0.01	0.02	0.03	0.04	0.05	0.06	0.07	0.08	0.09
0.00	50.00	50.40	50.80	51.20	51.60	51.99	52.39	52.79	53.19	53.59
0.10	53.98	54.38	54.78	55.17	55.57	55.96	56.36	56.75	57.14	57.53
0.20	57.93	58.32	58.71	59.10	59.48	59.87	60.26	60.64	61.03	61.41
0.30	61.79	62.17	62.55	62.93	63.31	63.68	64.06	64.43	64.80	65.17
0.40	65.54	65.91	66.28	66.64	67.00	67.36	67.72	68.08	68.44	68.79
0.50	69.15	69.50	69.85	70.19	70.54	70.88	71.23	71.57	71.90	72.24
0.60	72.57	72.91	73.24	73.57	73.89	74.22	74.54	74.86	75.17	75.49
0.70	75.80	76.11	76.42	76.73	77.03	77.34	77.64	77.94	78.23	78.52
0.80	78.81	79.10	79.39	79.67	79.95	80.23	80.51	80.78	81.06	81.33
0.90	81.59	81.86	82.12	82.38	82.64	82.89	83.15	83.40	83.65	83.89
1.00	84.13	84.38	84.61	84.85	85.08	85.31	85.54	85.77	85.99	86.21
1.10	86.43	86.65	86.86	87.08	87.29	87.49	87.70	87.90	88.10	88.30
1.20	88.49	88.69	88.88	89.07	89.25	89.44	89.62	89.80	89.97	90.15
1.30	90.32	90.49	90.66	90.82	90.99	91.15	91.31	91.47	91.62	91.77
1.40	91.92	92.07	92.22	92.36	92.51	92.65	92.79	92.92	93.06	93.19
1.50	93.32	93.45	93.57	93.70	93.82	93.94	94.06	94.18	94.30	94.41
1.60	94.52	94.63	94.74	94.85	94.95	95.05	95.15	95.25	95.35	95.45
1.70	95.54	95.64	95.73	95.82	95.91	95.99	96.08	96.16	96.25	96.33
1.80	96.41	96.49	96.56	96.64	96.71	96.78	96.86	96.93	97.00	97.06
1.90	97.13	97.19	97.26	97.32	97.38	97.44	97.50	97.56	97.62	97.67
2.00	97.73	97.78	97.83	97.88	97.93	97.98	98.03	98.08	98.12	98.17
2.10	98.21	98.26	98.30	98.34	98.38	98.42	98.46	98.50	98.54	98.57
2.20	98.61	98.65	98.68	98.71	98.75	98.78	98.81	98.84	98.87	98.90
2.30	98.93	98.96	98.98	99.01	99.04	99.06	99.09	99.11	99.13	99.16
2.40	99.18	99.20	99.22	99.25	99.27	99.29	99.31	99.32	99.34	99.36
2.50	99.38	99.40	99.41	99.43	99.45	99.46	99.48	99.49	99.51	99.52
2.60	99.53	99.55	99.56	99.57	99.59	99.60	99.61	99.62	99.63	99.64
2.70	99.65	99.66	99.67	99.68	99.69	99.70	99.71	99.72	99.73	99.74
2.80	99.74	99.75	99.76	99.77	99.77	99.78	99.79	99.79	99.80	99.81
2.90	99.81	99.82	99.83	99.83	99.84	99.84	99.85	99.85	99.86	99.86
3.00	99.87	99.87	99.87	99.88	99.88	99.89	99.89	99.89	99.90	99.90
3.10	99.90	99.91	99.91	99.91	99.92	99.92	99.92	99.92	99.93	99.93
3.20	99.93	99.93	99.94	99.94	99.94	99.94	99.94	99.95	99.95	99.95
3.30	99.95	99.95	99.95	99.96	99.96	99.96	99.96	99.96	99.96	99.97
3.40	99.97	99.97	99.97	99.97	99.97	99.97	99.97	99.97	99.97	99.98
−3.40	0.03	0.03	0.03	0.03	0.03	0.03	0.03	0.03	0.03	0.02
−3.30	0.05	0.05	0.05	0.04	0.04	0.04	0.04	0.04	0.04	0.03
−3.20	0.07	0.07	0.06	0.06	0.06	0.06	0.06	0.05	0.05	0.05
−3.10	0.10	0.09	0.09	0.09	0.08	0.08	0.08	0.08	0.07	0.07
−3.00	0.14	0.13	0.13	0.12	0.12	0.11	0.11	0.11	0.10	0.10
−2.90	0.19	0.18	0.18	0.17	0.16	0.16	0.15	0.15	0.14	0.14
−2.80	0.26	0.25	0.24	0.23	0.23	0.22	0.21	0.21	0.20	0.19
−2.70	0.35	0.34	0.33	0.32	0.31	0.30	0.29	0.28	0.27	0.26
−2.60	0.47	0.45	0.44	0.43	0.41	0.40	0.39	0.38	0.37	0.36
−2.50	0.62	0.60	0.59	0.57	0.55	0.54	0.52	0.51	0.49	0.48
−2.40	0.82	0.80	0.78	0.75	0.73	0.71	0.69	0.68	0.66	0.64
−2.30	1.08	1.04	1.02	0.99	0.96	0.94	0.91	0.89	0.87	0.84

Table A.4 (*Continued*)

z	\multicolumn{10}{c}{$100\Phi(Z)$}
	0.00	0.01	0.02	0.03	0.04	0.05	0.06	0.07	0.08	0.09
−2.20	1.39	1.36	1.32	1.29	1.26	1.22	1.19	1.16	1.13	1.10
−2.10	1.79	1.74	1.70	1.66	1.62	1.58	1.54	1.50	1.46	1.43
−2.00	2.28	2.22	2.17	2.12	2.07	2.02	1.97	1.92	1.88	1.83
−1.90	2.87	2.81	2.74	2.68	2.62	2.56	2.50	2.44	2.39	2.33
−1.80	3.59	3.52	3.44	3.36	3.29	3.22	3.14	3.07	3.01	2.94
−1.70	4.46	4.36	4.27	4.18	4.09	4.01	3.92	3.84	3.75	3.67
−1.60	5.48	5.37	5.26	5.16	5.05	4.95	4.85	4.75	4.65	4.55
−1.50	6.68	6.55	6.43	6.30	6.18	6.06	5.94	5.82	5.71	5.59
−1.40	8.08	7.93	7.78	7.64	7.49	7.35	7.22	7.08	6.94	6.81
−1.30	9.68	9.51	9.34	9.18	9.01	8.85	8.69	8.53	8.38	8.23
−1.20	11.51	11.31	11.12	10.93	10.75	10.56	10.38	10.20	10.03	9.85
−1.10	13.57	13.35	13.14	12.92	12.71	12.51	12.30	12.10	11.90	11.70
1.00	15.87	15.62	15.39	15.15	14.92	14.69	14.46	14.23	14.01	13.79
−0.90	18.41	18.14	17.88	17.62	17.36	17.11	16.85	16.60	16.35	16.11
−0.80	21.19	20.90	20.61	20.33	20.05	19.77	19.49	19.22	18.94	18.67
−0.70	24.20	23.89	23.58	23.27	22.97	22.66	22.36	22.06	21.77	21.48
−0.60	27.43	27.09	26.76	26.43	26.11	25.78	25.46	25.14	24.83	24.51
−0.50	30.85	30.50	30.15	29.81	29.46	29.12	28.77	28.43	28.10	27.76
−0.40	34.46	34.09	33.72	33.36	33.00	32.64	32.28	31.92	31.56	31.21
−0.30	38.21	37.83	37.45	37.07	36.69	36.32	35.94	35.57	35.20	34.83
−0.20	42.07	41.68	41.29	40.90	40.52	40.13	39.74	39.36	38.97	38.59
−0.10	46.02	45.62	45.22	44.83	44.43	44.04	43.64	43.25	42.86	42.47
−0.00	50.00	49.60	49.20	48.80	48.40	48.01	47.61	47.21	46.81	46.41

assumes a value located within the interval defined by the mean value ± 3 standard deviations, i.e., within the interval $[10 - 3 \cdot 2, 10 + 3 \cdot 2] = [4, 16]$. Using the transformation $Z = \frac{X-10}{2}$ we obtain a new random variable that follows a standardised Gaussian distribution. The probability that X will assume a value within the interval $[4,16]$ is equal to the probability that Z will assume a value within the interval $[\frac{4-10}{2}, \frac{16-10}{2}] = [-3, 3]$. This probability is equal to 1 minus the probability that Z will assume a value outside the interval, i.e., $1 - (P(Z \geq 3) + P(Z \leq -3)) = 1 - (0.00135 + 0.00135) = 0.9973$ (see the previous example). Therefore, the probability that a random variable that follows a Gaussian distribution will assume a value within the interval, mean value ± 3 standard deviations, is equal to 0.9973. The probability that it will assume a value outside this interval is: $0.00135 + 0.00135 = 0.0027$.

Estimates Based on a sample comprising n independent values of a random variable that follows a Gaussian distribution, the mean value of this distribution is estimated using the estimator

$$\overline{X} = \frac{\sum\limits_{i=1}^{n} X_i}{n} \qquad (A.21)$$

where x_i is the ith observation in the sample. This estimator is unbiased.

$$S^2 = \frac{\sum\limits_{i=1}^{n} (X_i - \overline{X})^2}{n - 1} \qquad (A.22)$$

is an estimator of the variance, σ^2. This estimator is also unbiased. By contrast, S is a biased estimator of σ. However, when n, the sample size, approaches infinity, the bias approaches 0. The bias of the estimated standard deviation based on a small sample may be adjusted. A quantity c_4, the value of which depends on the sample size n, is used. Its value for various values of n may be found in Table 1.1. The adjusted estimate of σ is $\frac{S}{c_4}$.

Example A.12

A sample consists of 6 independent observations of a random variable that follows a Gaussian distribution. The standard deviation of the sample is 0.334. Therefore, the unbiased estimate of the standard deviation of the Gaussian distribution (σ) is $\hat{\sigma} = \frac{0.334}{c_4}$. The value of c_4 is found by entering Table 1.1 at $n = 6$. We find $c_4 = 0.9515$. The estimate is $\frac{0.334}{0.9515} = 0.351$.

The central limit theorem The Gaussian distribution is very applicable in practice due to the central limit theorem that may be phrased as follows: if a sequence of n independent random variables is added, the distribution of their average (and also their sum) will converge towards a Gaussian distribution when n converges towards infinity. In practice, this implies that the average, or a sum of independent observations will follow a Gaussian distribution as long as the number of terms (n) is sufficiently large. What a sufficiently large number is, depends on the circumstances.

Example A.13

Figure A.1 shows the distribution of the physiological score of 870 surgical patients. Clearly, the distribution does not follow the Gaussian distribution that is symmetrical and bell shaped. On the contrary, it is markedly skewed to the right. We conduct three experiments. In the first one, the material is divided into groups of consecutive patient values, each comprising five values, and the mean value of the physiological scores is calculated for each group. Each of the following two experiments is a repetition of the first one, except that 10 patients are included per group in the second experiment and 15 in the third one.

Figures A.4 (a) through (c) show the histograms of the mean values of these experiments. In this experiment it was necessary to use a value of n that is larger than 10 in order to obtain a distribution with a shape, which approximates the symmetrical form of the Gaussian distribution.

Testing if a distribution is Gaussian The use of the Gaussian (normal) distribution is very common, and many statistical methods are based on the assumption that the data follow a Gaussian distribution. Therefore, it is important to be able to assess the validity of this assumption in practice. Most statistical software packages include several tools that may be used. The normal probability plot is an example of a graphical assessment. If the underlying population is normally distributed, the graph will be a straight line. In addition to the graph, several statistical tests for departures from normality exist. One test is called the Shapiro–Wilks W test [3]. It uses a measure of the straightness of the normal probability plot, and small values indicate departure from normality. There are other tests including one for skewness that tests if the distribution is symmetrical, and one for kurtosis that tests if the distribution is more, or less peaked than the Gaussian distribution [4].

Example A.14

Figure A.5 (a) depicts a normal probability plot of the cumulative relative frequency of the physiological scores of the mentioned 870 surgical

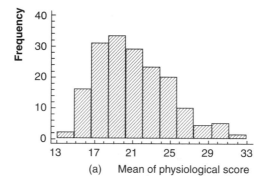

(a)   Mean of physiological score

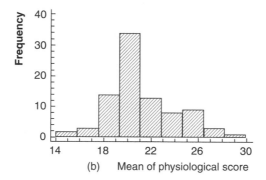

(b)   Mean of physiological score

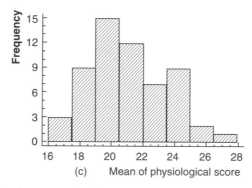

(c)   Mean of physiological score

Figure A.4   (a) The frequency distribution of the mean of the physiological score for $n = 5$. (b) The frequency distribution of the mean of the physiological score for $n = 10$. (c) The frequency distribution of the mean of the physiological score for $n = 15$.

patients. Figures A.5 (b) and (c) show the corresponding distributions of the mean values of samples comprising 10 and 15 patient values, respectively. In the first case (see Figure A.5 (a)), the accordance between the data and the theoretical straight line is indeed very poor. When the

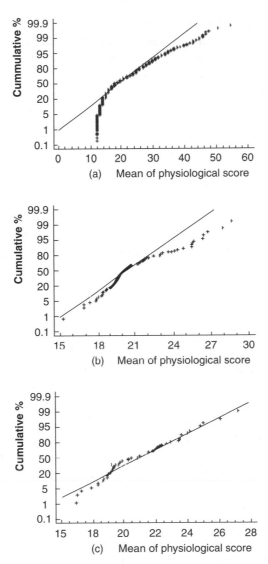

Figure A.5 (a) The cumulative relative frequency distribution of the physiological score, depicted in a Gaussian probability co-ordinate system. (b) The cumulative relative frequency distribution of the mean of the physiological score for $n = 10$, depicted in a Gaussian probability co-ordinate system. (c) The cumulative relative frequency distribution of the mean of the physiological score for $n = 15$, depicted in a Gaussian probability co-ordinate system.

sample size is 10 (Figure A.5 (b)), the accordance is considerably better, but still not quite satisfying. However, when $n = 15$, it is quite satisfying (Figure A.5 (c)). Since a graphical analysis is more or less subjective, it should be supplemented by statistical tests of the Gaussian hypothesis, e.g., the Shapiro–Wilks W test and the tests for skewness and kurtosis. The distribution of the original data as well as that of the means for $n = 10$ did not pass the Shapiro–Wilks W test for normality. However, the distribution of the means for $n = 15$ passed all tests. Therefore, in this example it is necessary to use a mean of 15 observations or perhaps slightly less before the distribution of the mean becomes Gaussian.

A.4 USING THE DATA

The data of a random sample obtained from a population may be used to calculate estimates of the parameters characterising the probability distribution generating the sample and to test various hypotheses about them.

A.4.1 Estimates

If samples are selected repeatedly from a population, and each sample is used to calculate an estimate, e.g., of the mean of the population, we obtain a distribution of sample estimates. Each of these estimates may be considered a sample from the unknown distribution of the population of all possible sample estimates, i.e., the distribution of the estimator.

This idea is exemplified in Figure A.6. If each sample consists of a single observation ($n = 1$) selected from a continuous distribution, e.g., a Gaussian one, the estimator of the mean of this distribution is the observation itself (use Equation (A.21) for $n = 1$). Therefore, the theoretical distribution of the estimator is identical to the distribution from which the sample was taken (see Figure A.6 first and second frame, respectively).

If the sample consists of n observations ($n > 1$), the estimator of the mean of the distribution is the mean of the sample values according to Equation (A.21). It may be shown: (1) that the theoretical distribution of the estimator of the mean is Gaussian if the original distribution, from which the sample was taken, is Gaussian; (2) that the distribution of the estimator has the same mean as the original distribution; and (3) has a standard deviation which is equal to that of the original distribution (σ) divided by $\sqrt{n}$ (see Figure A.6 third and fourth frame, respectively). Even if the original distribution is non-Gaussian, the distribution of the estimator of the mean is still Gaussian, provided n is sufficiently large. This follows from the central limit theorem [5].

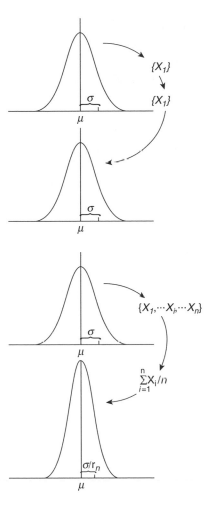

Figure A.6 Gaussian distribution with mean μ and standard deviation σ (first and third frames). Second and fourth frame show the distribution of the estimator of μ when the sample size (n) is 1 (second frame) and when $n > 1$ (fourth frame). The distributions of the estimators are Gaussian with mean $= \mu$ and standard deviation $= \frac{\sigma}{\sqrt{n}}$.

The distribution of other estimators, e.g., the estimator of the standard deviation of the original distribution, may be derived in an analogous way, using various types of statistical reasoning that may be found in most of the major statistical textbooks (see, e.g., [5]). The point is that the estimator itself follows a probability distribution, the precise nature of which depends on the original distribution from which the sample was taken and the sample size. The probability distribution of an estimator may often be characterised by a mean value and a standard deviation, as most other probability distributions.

A.4.2   Confidence Intervals

Using the standard deviation of the distribution of an estimator, also called the standard error, one may calculate a confidence interval for the parameter estimated. A confidence interval for a parameter is an interval calculated from the values of the sample, so that one has a specified certainty that the value of the parameter is contained within this interval. For example, a 95 % confidence interval is an interval that contains the parameter value with a 95 % certainty. The 95 % is referred to as the confidence level of the confidence interval. Imagine, that one selects a very large number of samples from some population and each time calculates the 95 % confidence interval of a parameter, for instance the mean value. We may then assume that the unknown parameter is contained within 95 % of these intervals. Loosely stated, the probability that an unknown parameter is contained within a specified 95 % confidence interval is 95 %. For a given level of confidence, the larger the standard deviation of the distribution of the estimator is, the wider the confidence interval.

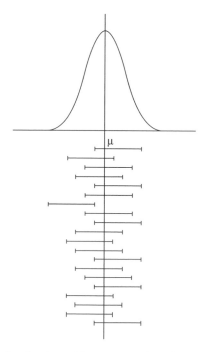

Figure A.7   Gaussian distribution with mean μ. Below the distribution are shown the 95 % confidence intervals of the mean (μ) computed from 20 samples. All, except one, contain the parameter μ.

Figure A.7 shows an invented example. At the top, a population of possible measurement values is shown. Below this distribution, 20 confidence intervals of the mean are shown. As expected, the mean value of the distribution is contained within 19 (95 %) of these intervals. Only one (5 %) of the samples, from which the intervals have been computed, is so extreme that the mean of the distribution is not contained within the 95 % confidence interval.

A.4.2.1 Calculating a confidence interval

When calculating a confidence interval for the mean or some other parameter, one usually needs the estimated value (E) of this parameter, the estimated standard deviation, which is often referred as standard error (S_E), and a quantity, such as t, given in Table A.5. The quantity required depends on the probability distribution of the estimator. If the random variable is normally distributed the value of the quantity typically depends on the degrees of freedom of s_E^2, the level of confidence, and whether one requires a one-sided or a two-sided interval.

Table A.5 Table of t values used when calculating a confidence interval of the mean. It is assumed that the sample data follow a Gaussian distribution.

Degrees of freedom	Level of confidence				
	Two-sided 80.0 % One-sided 90.0 %	90.0 % 95.0 %	95.0 % 97.5 %	98.0 % 99.0 %	99.0 % 99.5 %
1	3.078	6.314	12.706	31.821	63.657
2	1.886	2.920	4.303	6.965	9.925
3	1.638	2.353	3.182	4.541	5.841
4	1.533	2.132	2.776	3.747	4.604
5	1.476	2.015	2.571	3.365	4.032
6	1.440	1.943	2.447	3.143	3.707
7	1.415	1.895	2.365	2.998	3.499
8	1.397	1.860	2.306	2.896	3.355
9	1.383	1.833	2.262	2.821	3.250
10	1.372	1.812	2.228	2.764	3.169
11	1.363	1.796	2.201	2.718	3.106
12	1.356	1.782	2.179	2.681	3.055
13	1.350	1.771	2.160	2.650	3.012
14	1.345	1.761	2.145	2.624	2.977
15	1.341	1.753	2.131	2.602	2.947
16	1.337	1.746	2.120	2.583	2.921
60	1.296	1.671	2.000	2.390	2.660
120	1.289	1.658	1.980	2.358	2.617
∞	1.282	1.645	1.960	2.326	2.567

Table A.5 may be used when one is calculating a confidence interval for the mean value of a Gaussian distribution. For example, entering the table at column 5, line 5 (5 degrees of freedom), one finds the number 3.365. This value may be used to calculate the upper and lower limit of a 98 % two-sided confidence interval or the lower or upper limit of a one-sided 99 % confidence interval. The probability, that the true mean value is contained within the two-sided interval, is 98 %, implying that the probability that it is not contained within the interval is $(100 - 98)\% = 2\%$. This means that the probability that the parameter is larger than the calculated upper limit is 1 % and that it is smaller than the lower limit is 1 %.

The confidence interval of the mean value The confidence interval of the mean value of a Gaussian distribution may be calculated from a random sample of n independent observations from the distribution as follows

1. $\bar{x}$ and s are computed using the data.
2. The standard error of the mean is estimated as:

$$s_{\bar{x}} = \frac{s}{\sqrt{n}} \tag{A.23}$$

3. t, corresponding to the desired confidence level and degrees of freedom of s, is found in Table A.5.
4. The two-sided confidence interval is calculated as $\bar{x} \pm t \cdot s_{\bar{x}}$.

Example A.15

A sample comprising seven measurements has a mean of 8.00 and a standard deviation of 4.08. We want to calculate the two-sided 95 % confidence interval of the mean. s^2 has $n - 1 = 7 - 1 = 6$ degrees of freedom. For two-sided 95 % confidence intervals and 6 df, $t = 2.447$ (see Table A.5). The standard deviation of the mean is

$$\frac{s}{\sqrt{n}} = \frac{4.08}{\sqrt{7}} = 1.542$$

(see Equation (A.23)). Therefore, the confidence interval is $8.00 \pm 2.447 \cdot 1.542 = [4.23, 11.77]$.

Example A.16

In the previous example, had we wanted to calculate a one-sided 95 % confidence interval with an upper limit, we should have looked for the entry in Table A.5, corresponding to a 95 % one-sided confidence interval and 6 df. We find the value 1.943. The upper 95 % limit is $8.00 + 1.943 \cdot 1.542 = 11.00$. The limit of the corresponding one-sided confidence interval with a lower limit is $8.00 - 1.943 \cdot 1.542 = 5.00$.

A.4.3   Testing a Hypothesis

We may have some preconceived notion about the parameters of a population. For instance, assume that in previous investigations 50 years ago it was found that the average height of Danish males was 1.77 metre. We want to test the hypothesis that this is still the case. So we take a random sample from the population of Danish males and measure the heights of these males. To test a hypothesis based on a random sample, one postulates that the observations obtained are generated by a probability distribution the specifics of which depend on the stated hypothesis. In the example the hypothesis would be that the population of Danish males has a mean value equal to 1.77 metre. If the sample belongs to a category of extreme samples, which have a combined probability (α) of being selected that is very small if the hypothesis is true, the hypothesis is rejected. In this example, it might be samples with a mean larger than 1.95 metre or smaller than 1.59 metre. How small the probability, α (the level of significance of the test) should be, must be specified in advance. Usually α is set to 0.05 or 0.01. In other words, prior to the test, a region of acceptance is calculated. If the test result falls outside this region, the hypothesis is rejected. In the invented example the region was 1.59 to 1.95 metre.

Example A.17

At a market place, a tombola is located inside one of the tents. On a signboard the owner of the tent brags, 'you can't help winning a really excellent bottle of red wine if you draw a ticket from the tombola at the price of one dollar'. Immediately prior to the opening of the market place, the owner has placed 500 prize tickets in the tombola on each of which is written, 'Congratulations, you have just won a bottle of vintage red wine. Pursue your luck and buy another ticket'. The tent owner has asked his assistant to add an additional 4500 losing tickets to the 500 prize tickets. On each of them is written, 'you have been extremely unlucky. Please try once more'. The assistant, who had been testing a couple of bottles prior to his arrival at the market place, adds the additional 4500 tickets that he has brought with him. After having shuffled the tickets, he begins to doubt if the tickets he brought with him were losing tickets, a mixture of losing tickets and prize tickets, or even worse only prize tickets. He tells this to the tent owner who now has to decide if he should pack his things and return home or continue the tombola.

He hypothesises that all tickets are losing tickets, i.e., that the resulting mixture of tickets includes $\frac{500}{4500+500} = 10\,\%$ prize tickets which is suitable since the red wine was bought at Kmart, at two dollars a bottle. He wants to test this hypothesis, using a level of significance of 1 % or less. The alternative to his hypothesis is that the percentage is larger than 10 %. To test his hypothesis, he selects a random sample, comprising five tickets, from the tombola and notes their types (prize or losing tickets). If the hypothesis is true, the number of prize tickets in the sample follows a binomial distribution with parameters n and p, where p is the probability of selecting a prize ticket and n is the sample size. According to his hypothesis, there are 10 % prize tickets in the tombola. Hence $p = 0.1$ under the hypothesis. There are six possible outcomes of the test sampling: 0, 1, 2, 3, 4, or 5 prize tickets in the sample.

He defines a random variable, X that assumes a value equal to the number of prize tickets in the sample. He calculates the probability that X assumes a specified value x, using the formula

$$\frac{5!}{x!(5-x)!} \cdot 0.1^x \cdot 0.9^{(5-x)}$$

(see Equation (A.10)) to obtain $P(X = 0) = 0.59049$, $P(X = 1) = 0.32805$, $P(X = 2) = 0.0729$, $P(X = 3) = 0.0081$, $P(X = 4) = 0.00045$, and $P(X = 5) = 0.00001$.

The more prize tickets the sample contains, the more unlikely is the result, according to his hypothesis. If the hypothesis is true, the probability that the sample will contain three or more prize tickets is $0.0081 + 0.00045 + 0.00001 = 0.0086$ or 0.86 %. Therefore, he decides to reject the hypothesis if the sample contains three or more prize tickets. His region of acceptance is 0, 1, or 2 prize tickets in the sample.

Assume 4 of the 5 tickets are prize tickets. Since this is more than two, he rejects the hypothesis. The estimate of p is $\frac{4}{5} = 80\,\%$. That is, eight times as many as he had anticipated under the hypothesis.

If he gets a test value outside the region of acceptance, his postulate, that the hypothesis is wrong, is very well founded. By contrast, if the test value falls within the region of acceptance, his decision to accept the hypothesis may be less well founded. The cause of this is that the probability of obtaining a value within the region of acceptance may be quite high even if the hypothesis is wrong. For instance, if the true percentage of prize tickets is 20 % instead of 10 %, the probability of detecting it is actually less than 10 %. That is, the probability that the sample mean falls within the acceptance region is larger than 90 %. This weakness may be remedied if the size of the sample is increased, so that the number of possible outcomes increases.

A.4.4   Using a Confidence Interval to Test a Hypothesis

Testing a hypothesis using a specified level of significance and calculating a confidence interval with a specified level of confidence are two sides of the same matter. This is illustrated in the following example.

Example A.18

Following many disappointments, the regular customers of a middle-sized pub on the outskirts of London have decided to sue Brewery X. The plaintiffs claimed that the brewery was using misleading packaging for its products. This brewery had just introduced a new brand of beer. According to the label on the bottle it was supposed to contain half a litre. Brewery X claimed that the average volume per bottle in the local storage of beers of the mentioned brand was 500 ml. The regulars were allowed to select a reasonably sized random sample of bottles from the storage. Before the content of a bottle was drunk, the number of milli-litres contained within the bottle was first measured. An impartial person, jointly selected by Brewery X and the regulars of the pub, made these measurements. Based on the measurements, a 95 % confidence interval of the mean volume per bottle was calculated. This interval was [420 ml, 467 ml].

On these grounds Brewery X was sentenced to pay the expenses of the trial and in addition 10 cases of beer to each regular, 'as compensation for humiliation and pain', as the judge expressed it. Here is an extract of the judge's charge to the jury before they were considering the verdict and subsequently passing the sentence: '... if the mean volume is 500 ml, a 95 % confidence interval will not include this value in 5 % of the cases.' (Here the judge reviewed the definition of a confidence interval (see Section A.4.2, Figure A.7)) 'Therefore, if 500 ml is not contained in the confidence interval, we have obtained a sample that we would only obtain in 5 % of the cases if the hypothesis were true. Consequently it must be rejected...'.

To test the hypothesis that a parameter has a given value b, we select a sample from the population and calculate a $(1 - \alpha)$ confidence interval for the parameter, where α is the significance level chosen. If b is contained within the interval, the hypothesis is accepted; if not, it is rejected. If the level of significance is, e.g., 5 %, the confidence level should be 95 %. A one-sided confidence interval is relevant if a single alternative to the hypothesis can be specified (see Example A.17).

REFERENCES

[1] Barnett V, and Lewis T. Outliers in Statistical Data. John Wiley and Sons Ltd, Chichester, 1978.

[2] Copeland GP, Jones D, and Walters M. POSSUM: a scoring system for surgical audit. Br J Surg 1991; 78:356–60.

[3] Madansky A. Prescriptions for Working Statisticians. Springer-Verlag, New York, 1988.

[4] D'Agostino RB, and Stephens MA. Goodness-of-Fit Techniques. Butterworth and Co, London, 1986.

[5] Hald A. Statistical Theory with Engineering Applications. John Wiley and Sons Ltd, London, 1960.

Appendix B – $\overline{X}$ and S chart with variable sample size

When the sample size varies, $\hat{\mu}$ and $\overline{S}$ as estimators of μ and σ are calculated using weighted sample values as given in Equations (2.45) and (2.46)

$$\hat{\mu} = \frac{\sum_{i=1}^{k} n_i \overline{X}_i}{\sum_{i=1}^{k} n_i} \tag{B.1}$$

where $\overline{X}_i$ is the mean of the ith sample, n_i its size, and k the number of samples, and

$$\overline{S} = \sqrt{\frac{\sum_{i=1}^{k} S_i^2 (n_i - 1)}{\sum_{i=1}^{k} (n_i - 1)}} \tag{B.2}$$

where S_i is the standard deviation of the ith sample. The control limits of the $\overline{X}$ chart for the ith sample are given by

$$\hat{\mu} \pm 3 \frac{\overline{S}}{\sqrt{n_i}} \tag{B.3}$$

Statistical Development of Quality in Medicine   P. Winkel and N. F. Zhang
© 2007 John Wiley & Sons, Ltd

It can be shown that

$$\overline{S} = \frac{\sigma \chi_{h-1}}{\sqrt{h-1}} \tag{B.4}$$

where χ_h is a Chi statistic with degrees of freedom given by $h = \sum_{i=1}^{k} n_i - k + 1$ and σ is the standard deviation of X. It can be shown that

$$E[\overline{S}] = \frac{\sigma E[\chi_{h-1}]}{\sqrt{h-1}} = \sigma c_4(h) \tag{B.5}$$

with

$$c_4(h) = \sqrt{\frac{2}{h-1}} \frac{\Gamma\left(\frac{h}{2}\right)}{\Gamma\left(\frac{h-1}{2}\right)} \tag{B.6}$$

The factor $c_4(h)$ is the same as c_4 as given in Equation (2.17). The index h is used to emphasize that $c_4(h)$ is a function of h, which in the original definition in Equation (2.17) is the sample size. Thus, $\overline{S}$ is a biased estimator of σ and from (2.19)

$$\hat{\sigma} = \frac{\overline{S}}{c_4(h)} \tag{B.7}$$

is an unbiased estimator of σ. From (B.3), control limits of the $\overline{X}$ chart for the ith sample are given by Equation (2.47).

For the S chart, we plot the statistic S_i. The control limits are given by

$$E[\overline{S}_i] \pm 3\sqrt{\operatorname{Var}[\overline{S}_i]} \tag{B.8}$$

It is well known that

$$E[\overline{S}_i] = c_4(n_i)\sigma \tag{B.9}$$

and

$$\operatorname{Var}[\overline{S}_i] = (1 - c_4^2(n_i))\sigma^2 \tag{B.10}$$

Since $E[\overline{S}_i]$ depends on n_i, there is no central straight line for the S chart. The central point for the ith sample is at $E[\overline{S}_i]$, which from (B.9) and (B.7) is estimated by

$$c_4(n_i)\,\frac{\overline{S}}{c_4(h)}$$

as given in Equation (2.48). The upper and lower control limits at the ith sample are given by Equations (2.49) and (2.50).

Appendix C – Moving Range Estimator of the Standard Deviation of an AR (1) Process

The random variables X_j and X_{j-1} are Gaussian distributed with the same mean and variance, σ^2. Let $Y_j = X_j - X_{j-1}$, which is also Gaussian distributed with zero mean. Since $\{X_j; j = 1, 2, \ldots\}$ is an AR(1) process with parameter ϕ, from the properties of AR(1) processes in Section 4.1.2, $\rho(1) = \phi$. From Equation (4.3), the variance of Y_j, $j = 1, 2, \ldots$ is

$$\mathrm{Var}[Y_j] = 2\sigma^2 - 2\mathrm{Cov}[X_j, X_{j-1}]$$
$$= 2(1 - \phi)\sigma^2$$

From Patel and Read [1], $|Y_j|$ has a folded normal distribution with a mean of

$$E[|Y_j|] = \sqrt{\frac{2}{\pi}}\sqrt{\mathrm{Var}[Y_j]}$$
$$= \frac{2\sigma}{\sqrt{\pi}}\sqrt{1 - \phi}$$

Statistical Development of Quality in Medicine   P. Winkel and N. F. Zhang
© 2007 John Wiley & Sons, Ltd

From (4.12),

$$E[\hat{\sigma}_{MR}] = E\left[\sum_{j=2}^{k} \frac{|Y_j|}{d_2(k-1)}\right]$$

$$= \frac{E[|Y_j|]}{d_2}$$

$$= \sigma\sqrt{1-\phi}$$

since $d_2 = \frac{2}{\sqrt{\pi}} = 1.128$.

REFERENCES

[1] Patel JK, and Read CB. Handbook of the Normal Distribution. pp 33–4. Marcel Dekker, New York, 1982.

Index

Page references in **bold** indicate tables and those in *italics* indicate figures.